D0203041

Sexual Attraction

Sexual Attraction

The Psychology of Allure

James Giles

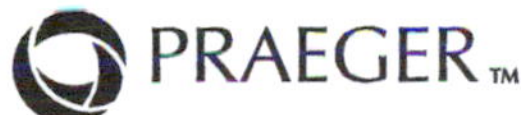

An Imprint of ABC-CLIO, LLC
Santa Barbara, California • Denver, Colorado

Copyright Acknowledgments

THE MAN COMING TOWARD YOU: A BOOK OF POEMS by Oscar Williams (1940), 13 lines from "Leg in the Subway." By permission of Oxford University Press.

"Strangers In The Night"
Adapted from A MAN COULD GET KILLED
Words by Charles Singleton and Eddie Snyder
Music by Bert Kaempfert

"Strangers In The Night"
Words by Charles Singleton and Eddie Snyder
Music by Bert Kaempfert

Library of Congress Cataloging-in-Publication Data

Giles, James, 1958–
Sexual attraction : the psychology of allure / James Giles.
pages cm
Includes bibliographical references and index.
ISBN 978-1-4408-3001-3 (hard copy : alk. paper) — ISBN 978-1-4408-3002-0 (ebook)
1. Sexual attraction. 2. Sex (Psychology) 3. Friendship. 4. Interpersonal relations. I. Title.
BF692.G537 2015
155.3'1—dc23 2015003882

ISBN: 978-1-4408-3001-3
EISBN: 978-1-4408-3002-0

19 18 17 16 15 1 2 3 4 5

This book is also available on the World Wide Web as an eBook.
Visit www.abc-clio.com for details.

Praeger
An Imprint of ABC-CLIO, LLC

ABC-CLIO, LLC
130 Cremona Drive, P.O. Box 1911
Santa Barbara, California 93116-1911

This book is printed on acid-free paper ∞

Manufactured in the United States of America

Contents

Preface vii

ONE: Interpersonal Attraction and Sexual Attraction 1
- Ways of Being Attracted to Other People 1
- Sexual Attraction and Physical Appearance 6
- Allure 25
- The Origins of Allure 33

TWO: Exchanging Glances 45
- Types of Strangers 45
- The Allure of Strangers 53
- Strangers in Dreams 71

THREE: Just Friends 83
- Friendship 83
- Cross-sex Friendship 99
- The Allure of Cross-sex Friends 118

FOUR: More than Just Friends 127
- Sexual Friendship 127
- The Place of Sex in Sexual Friendship 141
- The Allure of Sexual Friends 153

FIVE: It Turned Out So Right 165
- Romantic Attraction 165
- Lovers and Friends 180
- The Allure of Romantic Partners 189

SIX: With the Help of Helplessness 201
Notes 207
References 213
Index 225

Preface

This book is an attempt to give an account of the human experience of sexual attraction. Despite its fundamental role in everyday life, it is something that scholars have all but completely ignored. Various factors surrounding this experience have been studied, even in depth, but the experience itself remains an uncharted region of our existence. It is difficult to say why this is the case. One reason is probably that the study of human sexuality still remains an area filled with taboos. The study of sexuality has made dramatic progress in the last few decades, but for anyone familiar with this field it should be obvious that numerous topics are quickly skimmed over, discussions gingerly avoided, and distinctions not made. The reason for this is that to adequately discuss certain topics and make various distinctions in the field of sexuality one must explicitly address sexual experience and intimate activities. But this is just what people are reluctant to do. Consequently, in heeding the taboos one can only end up with an understanding that fails to grasp the richness of sexual experience. It is almost as if the researcher has popped into a room, taken a quick look around, and then quickly jumped out again. Not only does this create difficulties at the scientific and philosophical levels of understanding, but it reinforces the ancient Western prejudice that human sexuality is somehow a forbidden or at least disagreeable area. Since sexuality plays a fundamental role in our lives, paying respects to such a view can only be damaging to our well-being.

I first became aware of this problem in relation to sexual attraction when I was writing *The Nature of Sexual Desire*. For not only was it evident that scholars had for the most part neglected the nature of sexual desire, but no attempt had been made to distinguish it from sexual attraction. Indeed, the terms "sexual desire" and "sexual attraction" were often used indiscriminately, even in the same line, as if they referred to the same phenomenon. Yet after having worked on sexual desire it became clear to me that sexual attraction was a quite different, though related, phenomenon. It was my wanting to understand this related phenomenon of sexual attraction that led to the writing of this book. Consequently, this book can be seen as a sort of companion volume to *The Nature of Sexual Desire*. Both are explorations of distinct but related aspects of human sexuality.

This discovery, however, is not one that depends on anything more than looking directly at how we experience sexual attraction. There are, of course, other phenomena that surround and affect the experience, and these must be taken into consideration in order to fully understand sexual attraction. Nevertheless, it is vital that in doing so one does not lose sight of the core experience. In trying to maintain this awareness, I have found that the best way is to focus on people's descriptions of their experiences. This sort of approach has been called the phenomenological method and has been used widely in both philosophy and psychology. The problem is that there is little agreement on exactly what constitutes this method (other than the focus on experience) and how it is related to both other research methods and theoretical considerations. For these reasons I prefer to call the method I am using the experiential method, by which I mean simply that although data from other sources can play a supplemental role, the focus on experience is foremost and decisive. This method thus involves maintaining the primary focus on the subjective descriptions of experience. But it also involves supplementing these with both research findings from other approaches along with psychological theory and considerations from the philosophy of mind. Thus, if people's accounts of their experience of sexual attraction are either unclear or incomplete, I will then turn to research findings and theoretical considerations to help develop a clearer and more complete account. In all of this, however, the personal description plays the leading role. It is both the research from other approaches and theory that must accommodate the personal descriptions, not the other way around.

One of the methods I use in presenting the experiential material is to give the account from a first-person perspective. This is done to help focus attention on the subjective element in experience and present the material in a concrete way that makes it immediately accessible. A problem with doing this, however, is that a cursory or out-of-context reading might lead someone to think that I am describing my own personal experience rather than simply presenting my findings from a first-person point of view. This problem, however, can easily be solved by keeping this point in mind. I do, however, also refer to personal events that I myself have experienced. When I do so, it is explicitly stated and again should be clear from the context.

In getting access to these descriptions, I have used numerous sources, including unstructured interviews, informal discussions, discussions with my students, descriptions given in the research, film, erotic poetry, song lyrics, and other literature. Although some people might feel that such an approach is too wide in its focus, my feeling is that it gives us an insight into the nuances of a complex and overlooked experience by providing us with a diversity of angles from which to view it. The poet, it seems, is trying to capture a different aspect of sexual attraction than is the subject of an interview. With the poet it might be the awe or aesthetics of the experience that is foremost in his or her account. The interview subject, on the other hand, might attempt more to focus on what can be clearly expressed in a useful way to a researcher. Both angles provide different types of insight into a multifaceted process.

I have also tried to bring in data from a variety of both historical eras and cultures, wherever they are available. This has enabled me to show, I feel, that sexual attraction is a basic element in the human condition, rather than something that is merely a product or construction of culture. This was also facilitated by the fact that over the last years, when I was developing my ideas for this book, I was teaching at universities in several different cultures, including Micronesia, Hawaii, Australia, the United Kingdom, and Scandinavia, interacting with students from all over the world. Consequently, many of the interviews and discussions with my students involved people from diverse cultural backgrounds.

Using this approach, I have focused on giving an account of the experience of sexual attraction. This involves having to show how sexual attraction is fundamentally different from other forms of interpersonal attraction, how males and females respond to different aspects of each other, and how at the heart of sexual attraction lies the experience of allure—something that makes one feel helplessly drawn toward an intimate physical joining with the other person. Yet this experience is fundamentally entangled with the type of relationship in which it takes place. As a result, I also examine the main relationships we have—relationships to strangers, cross-sex friends, sexual friends, and types of romantic partners—in which sexual attraction tends to take place, and try to demonstrate how each of these relationships affects the subsequent experience of allure.

Nevertheless, sexual attraction is a phenomenon that appears in many more situations than I have been able to study here. Thus, there is sexual attraction in the atypical sexual variations, such as fetishism, transvestism, and zoophilia (sexual attraction to animals). But since the focus of this study is primarily heterosexual attraction between persons, I have had to leave these fascinating areas untouched. My feeling, however, is that the core of sexual attraction in such cases will also be explicable in terms of the psychology of allure. It is just that in these instances, what the individual is attracted to is a joining together with something that symbolizes another human being. Also, although I refer to homosexual attraction in various places, this is mainly for comparative purposes. Homosexual attraction shares much with heterosexual attraction but also differs in important ways. Consequently, a full study of homosexual attraction lies beyond the scope of this book. An inquiry into the complexity of homosexual attraction deserves a book of its own.

It is also worthwhile to say something about the notes used in this book. Throughout the text numbered notes appear. These, however, do not refer to any further discussions or other points, but only to the research and writings that support my claims. Consequently, while reading there is no need to stop each time one comes to a note and look it up unless one has a special interest in finding the relevant research or writings.

Finally, I should like to give my thanks to Ross Hughes for taking the time to read the manuscript and offer his helpful comments. Thanks are also due to the many people and especially my students who were kind enough to share with me their ideas on and experiences of sexual attraction.

ONE

Interpersonal Attraction and Sexual Attraction

WAYS OF BEING ATTRACTED TO OTHER PEOPLE

Sexual attraction plays a major role in most people's lives. Not only are people often concerned about their own sexual attractiveness, but also they are acutely aware of the sexual attractiveness of other people. Sexual attraction shows its importance in our lives by typically guiding us to those who become our sexual, romantic, or lifelong partners. But it also fills our awareness as we go about our daily lives. People we pass in the street, work colleagues, classmates, and family friends, all present themselves to our awareness in terms of their degree of sexual attractiveness.

This is not to say that people appear to us only in this way. Nor is it to say everyone is always trying to make himself or herself sexually attractive. It simply means that one of the basic ways in which we experience others is in terms of their sexual attractiveness. And this is something we do regardless of whether the other person wants us to or is even aware that we are doing it. This is, of course, also true for other types of human attraction, for sexual attraction shares much in common with them. The reason for this is that sexual attraction, in its most common variety, is a type of interpersonal attraction. There are, however, fundamental differences between sexual attraction and other ways of being attracted to people. Understanding the nature of these differences will help in getting clear about the nature of sexual attraction itself.

To start, it can be noted that interpersonal attraction is often thought of as any form of positive attitude or disposition toward another person. Apart from sexual attraction, this can take such forms as affiliation, liking, friendship, kinship, or love in all its varieties. An interesting feature about these forms of attraction is that they both overlap and disjoin in various ways. Affiliation, which is simply being attracted to someone in order to be in his or her presence, can also appear in liking. This is obvious because when I like someone, I often want to spend time with him or her. However, this need not be the case. I can like someone and yet feel no need to seek out the individual's company. This would seem especially so where the liking was of a mild degree. In such a case, I enjoy the person when I have a chance to be with him or her, say, at some form of social gathering. But when the meeting is over, I feel no need to seek further affiliation to the person. I enjoyed his or her company for the moment, now that moment is gone, and I return to my other concerns.

In the same way, there is no reason why affiliation need include liking. Often it does, but often it does not. Consider the case of someone who admires another person and so wants to spend time with that person, perhaps to learn from the person or perhaps just to be near him. In such a case the experience of liking might well be foreign to the experience of affiliation. Something like this seems to be going on with people who follow and seek out the company of high-status others or celebrities. One could even imagine a case where the admirer does not particularly like the admired person. Perhaps he knows things about the individual to whom he wants to be affiliated, things that he feels render that individual unlikable as a person. Nevertheless, he may still admire the person for other reasons and so seek affiliation to the person.

Similar things could be said about love and liking. For although people who are in love often like their beloved, again this need not always be the case. A person in the throes of romantic love might feel a dislike toward her beloved for numerous reasons: perhaps she feels he does not show her enough attention, perhaps she feels he shows too much attention to other women, or perhaps he is not interested in disclosing his feelings to her. All of this might make her feel a strong dislike toward him, even though at the same time she deeply loves him. It is important also to note that this need not be a temporary disliking. Instead, it might well be the essence of the relationship. This difference between love and liking is well captured in the lyrics of the song "You Really Got a Hold on Me" made popular by the Beatles. Here the singer explains, "I don't like you, but I love you," making a clear distinction between these two forms of attraction. Then, to explain further why he does not like her, and also to account for how this gets him to love her, he says, "You treat me badly, I love you madly."

Contrary to this, there are further types of interpersonal attraction that clearly do overlap. For example, friendship includes liking, while both friendship and love include the attraction of affiliation. Friendship includes liking simply because, in one way, friendship is a relationship of mutual liking between two individuals. The attraction in friendship is a liking toward someone who likes you back. The liking of friendship, however, is somewhat different from the liking that occurs outside of friendship. This is because in friendship, part of what we like about a friend is that the friend likes us back. This feature is lacking when one likes a person who is not one's friend. Still, the liking of a friend would seem to include the same sort of positive feeling and evaluation of someone who is liked, even though he or she is not a friend.

In the case of friendship and love, both include affiliation because both include, among other things, the desire to spend time with the other person. It is worth noting here that the attraction of friendship might even, at least in some cases, include attraction to things like the intelligence, financial resources, or athletic ability of the other person.[1] Since these features appear to be more like the stuff of affiliation, this also seems to indicate there can be an overlapping between the attraction of affiliation and attraction in some types of friendship.

Kinship is also an interpersonal relation that can include various forms of interpersonal attraction. It is not, however, in itself a form of interpersonal attraction but refers rather to familial relations between, say, parent and child or siblings (either biological or adoptive relations). Parents and children or siblings, for example, can like each other or have different sorts of love for each other and have each of these in various degrees of overlapping. But none of this need be the case. It is, however, only when there is some such positive attitude toward a family member that kinship can be considered a form of interpersonal attraction.

Another relation that needs to be mentioned here is that of physical attraction. This refers to the experience of finding another person's physical appearance to be aesthetically pleasing or attractive. This is something that is frequently discussed in the research on interpersonal attraction. There is, however, no clear agreement about how it fits into the general picture of interpersonal attraction. One of the main problems here seems to be that although it is often discussed as if it were a type of attraction—much like friendship and love are types of attraction—it seems more properly understood as a component of different forms of interpersonal attraction. For example, it is often pointed out that things like proximity, similarity, and physical attraction can affect interpersonal attraction.[2] Therefore, the closer and more similar someone is to another person, and the more physically attractive he is, the better the chances are that the other person will, for example, like him or seek out his friendship. This suggests that the element of physical attraction works as a component that influences different types of attraction, rather than its being a distinct type of attraction. Furthermore, if someone seeks out the company of another person merely because of the other person's physical attractiveness, this is simply a type of affiliation. As just mentioned, affiliation can be based on such things as admiration or the desire to be near someone for other reasons. One such reason can be the person's physical attractiveness.

Now, the fascinating thing about sexual attraction is that while other forms of attraction often depend on the attracted person knowing—or at least thinking that he or she knows—something about the personality, attitudes, or abilities of the person to whom he or she is attracted, sexual attraction does not. This is why, though a form of interpersonal attraction, sexual attraction cannot be explained in terms of the two-dimensional model that has been recently proposed for understanding interpersonal attraction generally. According to this model, an individual's attraction to another person is based on the individual's evaluation of both the other person's capacity to facilitate the observer's goals or needs and the other person's willingness to facilitate those goals or needs.[3] In other words, regardless of the type of attraction we feel to another individual, what motivates our attraction is, first, the idea that the individual has the capacity to give us what we want and, secondly, that the individual is willing to give us what we want.

Although this model might account for some forms of interpersonal attraction, when it comes to sexual attraction, it is unclear how either of the two dimensions works to create attraction. Considering the first dimension, it seems natural to ask how it is that, strictly on the basis of his or her physical appearance, a particular person is evaluated as having a capacity to facilitate one's goals or needs. For why should one person be evaluated as having a capacity to facilitate one's goals or needs in a way that another person is not? Since the "goal" of sexual attraction is a warm and intimate baring and caressing with another person's body, the question becomes "How can a person with one appearance facilitate this goal or need in a way that a person with another appearance cannot?" A woman, for example, might find a man sexually attractive particularly because of the shape of his face, color of his eyes, and his way of walking. But it is unclear why these particular features should be seen as giving the man a capacity to facilitate her goal of intimate baring and caressing or, say, having sexual intercourse with the man. Why could not a man who lacks these features, or even have features that she finds unattractive, equally well facilitate her goal?

Or imagine a man who finds a woman sexually attractive because of the length and texture of her hair, the smoothness of her skin, and the shape of her buttocks. Imagine also that his goal is specifically to have this woman perform fellatio on him. There is no evident reason why these particular features render this woman any better at facilitating his goal than another woman who lacks these features. Indeed, in both these cases it looks very much like the idea of the other person's capacity to facilitate the observer's goals or needs has little to do with the sexual attraction. Rather, the experience of sexual attraction simply asserts itself without any consideration of the attractive person's specific capacities to facilitate goals or needs.

And the same could be said concerning the second dimension, namely, the other person's willingness to facilitate those goals or needs. For plainly, sexual attraction has nothing to do with the idea that the other person is willing to facilitate such needs. This is obvious from the fact that we often find someone sexually attractive regardless of how we evaluate his or her willingness to facilitate our needs. Of course, the idea that the other person would be willing to facilitate one's specific sexual needs might add a further dimension or urgency to one's sexual attraction, but clearly it is not necessary. This is underlined by the fact that we can even find someone sexually attractive who shows a clear unwillingness to facilitate our needs.

It is because sexual attraction operates in this way that one can easily feel sexual attraction for a complete stranger. It is true that people, with little or no evidence, are quick to form impressions of strangers. Psychological mechanisms like stereotyping, forming a judgment on a single piece of evidence, or assumption of similarity (the assumption that someone must be similar to another person because of a minor feature they share in common) can all can play a role in our quickly attributing personality traits to someone we have seen for the first time.[4] I think, however, that such mechanisms play a negligible role in the initial experience of sexual attraction. For it is not that we first form an impression of a stranger and then, on the basis of that impression, find him or her sexually attractive. Rather, if impression formation does come into it, it seems we first find the stranger sexually attractive and then, on the basis of that attraction, form an impression of the person. Therefore, by the time we form the impression, we have already experienced sexual attraction for the person. No doubt such impressions can affect the initial sexual attraction by altering it in various ways. It would be wrong, however, to say they were essentially responsible for it.

SEXUAL ATTRACTION AND PHYSICAL APPEARANCE

But if our impression of a person is not necessary to engender sexual attraction, what, then, is it that leads to sexual attraction? The obvious answer is physical appearance. The reason for this is that sexual attraction is intimately tied to physical appearance, and the ability to note another person's physical appearance requires no foreknowledge about the individual's willingness to do anything nor about his or her interests or personality. Thus, for example, the stranger I see sitting in the airport waiting lounge immediately strikes me as sexually attractive simply because of her appearance: say, the shape of her mouth, the way her hair falls about her neck, the fullness of her hips and thighs, and the slenderness of her hands. Her personality, dispositions, and so forth are all unknown to me. Further, they are irrelevant as far as her immediate sexual attraction goes. Of course, I could try to speculate about her personality or her willingness to do various things for me, basing my speculations on her way of dressing or perhaps the book she is reading. But why would I engage in such speculations unless she first stirred my attraction? If she was someone I did not find sexually attractive, then for me, she would be just one more stranger in the crowd, and my gaze would have no doubt continued without taking any notice of her (unless something else about her roused my interest). It seems, therefore, that it would be the initial sexual attraction that led to my wondering about her other qualities, not my imagining of those qualities that led to my sexual attraction.

It is worth noting here, too, that physical appearance does not just refer to someone's static visual appearance, but also to the appearance of the person's body in motion and activities. Further, it does not just refer to the visual appearance that someone has to others, but also to the touch, taste, smell, and sound of the person. One woman, for example, refers to her sudden sexual attraction to a man saying, "I was sitting in the train on the way home when a man came and sat beside me. At first I didn't really notice him. But he smelled so good that I had to look up at him. And there sat the sweetest redheaded man smiling at me. As I got off the train I turned back and noticed he was still looking at me. I regret so much that I didn't say anything to him."[5] In this description of sexual attraction, there are four main physical features that seem to capture the woman's attention. These are his scent, his red hair, his smile, and his looking at her. Of these features, only the red hair refers to a static visual feature of the man, and it is not even clear if this is something that attracts her or merely something that she notices. The other physical features, which seem to have set her sexual attraction in motion, are his smell and his activities of smiling and looking at her.

One could ask, I suppose, whether smiling and looking at someone are more than merely physical activities. For smiling might be indicative of a friendly personality and looking at someone as showing interest. In this case, however, my guess would be that the smiling and looking are only sexually attractive because they are done by a good-smelling sweet redheaded man, that is, by a man with otherwise sexually attractive features. It was the man's scent, it should be noted, that first and powerfully caught the woman's attention.

In the same way it should be noted that the nonvisual physical activities of talking and walking are also powerful elements in sexual attraction. Males and females have distinct voice qualities with women's voices being higher pitched than men's. These differences are both obvious and sexually attractive for both sexes. Thus, females show a preference for low-pitched male voices,[6] while males find higher-pitched female voices attractive.[7] Interestingly enough, with women this preference might be correlated with overall size, with a larger woman preferring a lower-pitched voice.[8] This might well be because a lower-pitched male voice is typically indicative of a larger male, and women normally do not want to be larger or taller than their sexual partners. With men, there might also be limiting factors here; for although men are more attracted to higher-pitched female voices, female voices over a certain level of pitch (about 280 Hz) are judged to be less attractive. This might be because female voices with too high a pitch sound babyish and thus create an association with sexual immaturity (that is, with an immature body).[9]

Similarly, the way of walking can also be something that influences sexual attraction. Here, too, males and females have distinct behavioral features.[10] Men have more velocity, take longer strides, and make slower movements. They also have more head movement and upper-body side-sway. Women, on the other hand, take smaller steps and show quicker movements, more back arching, and more hip and buttock motion. Further, both men and women are very good at spotting these differences in gaits: individuals walking in the distance are normally quickly discerned to be male or female simply by their gait. This distinction, along with our sensitivity to it, enables walking to be an aspect of sexual attractiveness. Both these factors would seem to be among the main reasons for the widespread use of high heels by women, both in Western culture and beyond. High heels exaggerate the features of the female way of walking, making the woman seem more sexually attractive. Men (and women) watching representations of women walking in point-light displays—moving dots of light on a screen that represent the limbs of a walker—consistently rate women walking in high heels as more sexually attractive than women walking in flat shoes.[11] And both men and women do this even though they cannot see the high heels, for the type of shoes is not evident in the point-light display. It is not, therefore, the shoes themselves that are seen to increase their attractiveness, at least not in light-point displays. Moreover, it is well known that, in order to make themselves more sexually attractive, female models on the catwalk use a particular gait that, especially when done in high heels, further exaggerates the female walking style. They do this by swinging one foot in front of the other in order to increase the swinging of the hips and the motion in the buttocks.

It should be noted that various other cultures also have, in their own ways, attempted to exaggerate the female gait. In Japanese culture, for example, the traditional woman's kimono is worn in such a way that it restricts the woman's stride, thus making her take shorter steps. This effect is further enhanced by the use of high platform-like shoes worn especially by geishas and maikos (geishas in training), shoes that make the heel and ball of the foot hit the ground at the same time. It is these attempts to exaggerate the sexually attractive aspects of female walking that seem also to lie behind the development of many forms of female dancing. Thus, belly dancing with its hip shaking, ballet with its short steps (taken in invisible high heels), and even ladies' figure skating with its back arching (as in the layback and Biellmann spins) and outward-pushed buttocks (as in backward skating), are all exaggerations of female movements.

This discussion leads naturally to the role of clothing in creating sexual attraction. As everybody knows, clothing and other such accessories play a large part in enhancing sexual attraction. The reason for this is simply that clothing can be used to accentuate or decorate sexually attractive aspects of a person's physical appearance. Women's clothing that emphasizes the figure, buttocks, or breasts or that shows bare skin, or men's clothes that accentuate a man's slimness, flat stomach, or small buttocks, all work to draw attention to the contours of the body.

Clothing can also serve other social functions. It can, for example, imply something about the wearer's personality or social or economic status. Thus, dressing in a nonconforming way might be done to imply an exhibitionistic or rebellious disposition, or it might merely show a lack of value of social norms. Wearing clothes that are flaunted by a particular group or subculture can be a way of signaling that one wants to be seen as belonging to that group, whereas dressing in expensive or designer clothes may be an attempt to imply that one has wealth or status or that one is "in the know." Although clothes serving these functions—functions that do not direct attention to the body—might seem to influence sexual attraction, what they primarily influence, at least in the realm of interpersonal attraction, is attraction for other reasons. With men this seems especially true. As one woman put it, "While stylish wardrobes do boost attractiveness, it's only because they increase a man's cachet, not his raw handsomeness."[12] I shall come to these other reasons for attraction shortly.

The question of why sexual attraction has this basic connection to physical appearance should not be difficult to answer. One need simply note that sexual attraction involves the other person's body (or at least what one imagines is the other person's body). This is because the ultimate goal of sexual attraction is to bring one's own body into an intimate exchange of baring and caressing with the other person's body, even if, as I shall argue, for other reasons one chooses not to. Thus, in finding the woman in the airport lounge sexually attractive, I am immediately brought to the idea of her lips on mine, my fingers running through her hair and caressing her neck, her hips and thighs pressed up against me, and her hand clasping mine.

This, of course, is only one sort of intimate exchange of baring and caressing. Different people can have different ideas. One of my students, for example, a Japanese woman in her mid-20s, related how whenever she saw a man she found sexually attractive, she immediately thought of sinking her teeth into his lovely body, as she put it. Here the idea of baring and caressing takes the form of teeth pressing firmly into naked flesh, a form of erotic caressing that is also discussed in the *Kāma Sūtra*, the ancient Indian book on sex and love. It is perhaps worth noting that the idea of an intimate exchange through sinking teeth into an attractive person can be carried a step further to the idea of actually consuming the attractive person. In an advertisement for women's facials, for example, one cosmetic shop in Melbourne used the slogan "Skin good enough to eat," posted just under the photograph of a coyly smiling and sexually attractive woman (with apparently edible skin).[13]

But, one might ask, if sexual attraction is tied to physical appearance, why is it that sexual attraction seems often provoked by things that have little to do with physical appearance? Why, for example, do people sometimes seem sexually attracted to another person because of the person's possessions, status, or personality (which, as I suggested, clothes can be used to imply)? This is a complex question. I think, however, the answer lies in seeing that, in such cases, what the attracted person experiences is not really sexual attraction; it is foremost another form of attraction or at least is something that gets someone to view the person's appearance in a new way.

To see how this works, consider the situation in which a woman seems sexually attracted to a man because of his money or social status. This would seem to be a case in which a person is sexually attracted to another person regardless of his physical appearance. His possessions or status seem to somehow imbue him with sexual attractiveness that has little to do with his physical appearance.

The problem, however, is one could always raise the question of whether she is really sexually attracted to him. Might it not be that what she is really attracted to is his money and that her supposed sexual attraction is merely pretense, or even a self-deception, in order that she might be able to avail herself of his money? Or maybe she likes the idea that her own apparent attractiveness or status will appear to be enhanced when she is seen with him.

A good example of this can be seen in a popular Internet video entitled "Gold digger prank!" The video is a prank in which a hidden camera films a man (the prankster) who approaches a woman. He says that he was looking at her and finds her pretty, and asks if she would be interested in going out with him to dinner. She rebuffs him nonchalantly, saying she does not go out to dinner with people, and continues to walk away showing no interest in the man. When she notices, however, that he is getting into a luxury sports car to drive away, she suddenly stops and asks, "Is that your car?" When he replies that it is, she quickly changes her attitude to the man and says, "Well, I might be able to go out to dinner with you" and even suggests a nearby place where they could go.

Now, one could try to explain what is going on here by saying that even though the woman was not initially sexually attracted to the man, upon seeing his car she suddenly became attracted to him. But how could this happen? How could seeing the car suddenly make the man look sexually attractive? One answer might be that seeing the car enabled her to somehow focus on the man in a sharper way. Perhaps noticing the car made her look more closely at the man and got her to see sexually attractive features she had not noticed initially. But this seems unlikely; for in the video it is quite evident that it is the car that catches and holds her interest, not that the car directs her interest to the man.

A more likely explanation is that she does not, even upon seeing the car, find the man sexually attractive. Rather, upon seeing the car she suddenly sees the man as being affluent. She then also realizes that the man's sexual attraction to her implies that, were she to accept his offer, she might have access to the benefits of his affluence. Not only might this mean that she could be treated to expensive dinners and given expensive gifts, while being driven about in a fancy car, but also that being seen with him would increase her status as an attractive female. For why (her thinking might go) would a man with so much money, a man who could get many women, choose to be with her? The obvious reason must be that she is exceptionally attractive. This, she might imagine, is what other people would think.

In all of this it is instructive to note that no thought is given to the man's sexual attractiveness. The decision to accept the man's offer is based purely on the idea that the man owns a luxury sports car and all that it implies. This does not mean—and here is the important point—that the woman is not drawn into wanting to have sex with the man. For she can easily want to have sex with the man without feeling any sexual attraction to him. This is because sexual attraction is not the only reason for deciding to have sex with someone. In this example, the woman might well realize that, if she is to stay the course and get the benefits of the man's supposed wealth, then eventually she will probably have to have sex with him. And she might be willing to do this. Or rather than simply be willing to do it, she might actually want to have sex with the man. There are numerous possible reasons for this: she might feel that having sex with him would help secure his interest in her, that it would be a way of rewarding his interest in her, that it would prove he found her sexually attractive, and so on. Or again, she might simply be in the throes of self-deception. She might want to have sex with him in order to convince herself that she does actually find him sexually attractive (even though she does not) and so convince herself that she is not only interested in his money (which in fact she is). (Luckily, or perhaps unluckily, things never come to this and the man simply drives off without her, saying, "I don't like gold diggers.")

Although this is only one example—a woman showing apparent sexual attraction to a man because of his car—much of the argument is, I feel, applicable to other cases where things like possessions and status seem to lead to sexual attraction. In other words, what often appears to be sexual attraction to someone because of his possessions or status is not sexual attraction at all, but rather something like a pragmatic calculation based on other goals, or even self-deception. Therefore, such cases do not show that sexual attraction can operate without any concern for physical appearance. They only show that people can decide to pursue someone sexually or to have sex with someone for reasons other than sexual attraction, even though it is made to look like sexual attraction.

But what about the case where someone seems to find another person sexually attractive because of features of his or her personality, say, such things as kindness, warmth, or sense of humor? It sometimes seems, for example, that sexual attraction only develops after an individual gets to know something about the personality of the other person. Therefore, although an individual may notice the physical appearance of another person, in such a case it is not enough to lead to sexual attraction. Here sexual attraction only appears once the individual gets to experience the other person's personality. In such cases it looks again like sexual attraction is directed toward the individual's personality and has little connection to physical appearance.

There is, however, another explanation. This explanation is based on the well-known fact that the physical appearance of another person seems to change once we get to know the person better. Furthermore, it appears that as we start to like another person for his or her personality, the person seems to become better looking. There is even research that confirms this common experience. One study had two groups of subjects watch two different videos of the same professor talking to his students. In the "cold condition" video the professor was critical, unpleasant, and unkind to the students, while in the "warm" condition video he was supportive, encouraging, and kind. The subjects watching the "cold" condition video expressed a dislike for the professor, while the subjects watching the "warm" condition video liked the professor. The researchers then asked the subjects to evaluate the physical attractiveness of the professor. The results were that the subjects who disliked the professor rated him as being physically unattractive, while the subjects who liked him rated him as being more physically attractive.[14]

Further, just to make sure subjects were not influenced by the professor's physical expressions (which could be seen as part of his physical appearance), they then showed the two videos to a separate group of subjects, but this time without the sound. In this condition, the subjects did not like him more in the warm condition than in the cold condition, nor did they find him any more attractive in one condition than in the other. This showed that what was causing the first two groups of subjects to evaluate the professor's physical attractiveness differently was his apparent personality, not his physical expressions. Accordingly, it seems clear that how we come to feel about someone as a person affects our perception of the person's attractiveness.

Now, although the researchers did not distinguish between physical and sexual attractiveness, I think it likely that the perception of someone's sexual attractiveness would be affected in the same way. One cartoon I saw expressed this phenomenon by having a man say to a woman that when he was first in love with her, suddenly her eyes did not seem so close together. But since those early feelings have worn off, her eyes seemed to him close together again. It therefore appears that as we get to like someone of the opposite sex for his or her personality, at some point that person becomes sexually attractive to us, though this will naturally depend on the person already having certain features that we find more or less sexually attractive to begin with.

But if this is what happens, then in such cases it looks as though sexual attraction is not directed to the individual's personality after all, but rather to what the attracted person takes to be the attractive individual's physical appearance. The attractive individual's personality plays a role in sexual attraction only so far as it gets the attracted person to see the individual's physical appearance in a more attractive light. It is still, in the end, the physical appearance or apparent physical appearance that is the immediate cause of the observer's sexual attraction.

One could always object to this by saying that even though someone's physical appearance seems to become more sexually attractive to the person who starts liking her, this does not mean it is the physical appearance that is the cause of the sexual attraction. For maybe upon coming to like someone for her personality, one then becomes sexually attracted by her personality. This might well lead to a sexually enhanced perception of her physical appearance, but this would merely be an effect of the initial sexual attraction to her personality. In other words, it is still the personality that, in such cases, is the original cause of the sexual attraction.

The problem with this account, however, is that there is no reason to prefer it over the explanation that I have just presented. The view that sexual attraction is stimulated by physical appearance fits well with everyday experience. And in those other cases where sexual attraction seems to be provoked by things like money, cars, and other possessions, there is good reason to believe, as I have shown, that these are only cases of apparent sexual attraction where the attraction is really to something else. Since personality is, like money and possessions, also quite distinct from physical appearance, it seems likely that it is the apparently enhanced physical appearance (caused by the liking of the personality) that is the real cause of the sexual attraction.

But why, it could be asked, cannot someone be sexually attracted to an individual's personality? With a car or possessions, these seem quite distinct from an individual's physical appearance. So it is understandable that in such a case, what is involved is simply an interest in the car, not a sexual attraction to the car owner. But in the case of personality this is something that is not so distinct from the person's physical appearance. Personality is, after all, expressed by a physical body, and physical bodies have a physical appearance. Consequently, being sexually attracted to someone because of his or her personality might not be that distinct from being sexually attracted to someone because of his or her physical appearance.

Although this point has some truth to it, I think there still remains a significance difference between physical appearance and personality, at least as far as sexual attraction goes. Consider the case of someone who feels he is sexually attracted to the personality traits of ambitiousness, thoughtfulness, and creativity. The first thing to notice is that these personality traits can be displayed by people of widely different physical appearances, even appearances that the observer might find sexually repulsive. In such a case it would seem unlikely that the observer would, upon experiencing the personality traits, suddenly find the person sexually attractive. And if this is the case, then it seems unlikely that it is the personality traits that are the real basis of his sexual attraction. Of course, he might begin to like the individual as a person, enjoying her creativity, and so on. Further, he might even begin to consider her as a long-term partner, and even eventually want to have sex with her. But in none of these cases does this show that he is sexually attracted to her. For, as I have argued, all of this can take place in the absence of sexual attraction.

Maybe what is really important to someone is to have a sexual partner who shows specific personality traits. Also, maybe this person has been unable to find a partner who both is sexually attractive and has these personality traits. As a result, he may well be willing to accept a sexual partner he does not find sexually attractive as long as she has the desired personality traits. Finally, like the case of the woman whose real interest is the man's car, this person might even begin to deceive himself into believing that he finds his partner sexually attractive.

This points to what is wrong with much of the research that purports to show that while men are sexually attracted to physical appearance, women are sexually attracted to things like personality or status. For such research typically fails to distinguish between sexual attraction and attraction for other reasons. For example, in one review of research findings on "opposite-sex attraction" (that is, sexual attraction) to a stranger, it is concluded that men value physical attractiveness more than women do, and that women value (similarity of) personality more than men do. It is further concluded that women value similarity more than they value attractiveness.[15]

Yet no attempt is made to distinguish between immediate sexual attraction and attraction to a potential long-term partner. For the obvious question to ask is if the women in these studies are valuing similarity of personality over sexual attractiveness simply because they are considering the men they are judging as potential long-term partners. This is an obvious question because it makes sense that one might be attracted to similarity of personality when considering someone as a long-term partner. Even here, however, things are not so straightforward. For evidence suggests that although someone might initially be attracted to actual similarity in a potential partner, this is only when there has been little or no interaction. As the amount of interaction increases, the role of actual similarity decreases. In existing sexual relationships it might even play no role in attraction at all. What does play a role, however, is, perceived similarity.[16] So even though there may be little actual similarity between those in an existing relationship, there will tend to be perceived similarity. But where does this perceived similarity come from? One likely answer is that it comes from the initial sexual attraction. Therefore, rather than perceived similarity leading to sexual attraction, it could well be the other way around, namely, that it is sexual attraction that initially leads to perceived similarity.

Because of this, and because our societal norms tend to encourage women to think in terms of finding a long-term rather than short-term partner, it appears likely that the women in these studies would be thinking in terms of what is important in a long-term partner. This seems especially so when one notes that the studies in this review are all questionnaires or artificial experimental studies rather than real-life situations in which a person is confronted with a potential, actual sex partner. In such a situation it might well be that the sexual attractiveness of the potential partner would assert itself more immediately and more strongly, with other long-term considerations fading into the background.

Remarkably enough, this is just what happens in a well-known field study or "real-life" study of sexual attraction.[17] In this study university students were invited to a dance where they were randomly assigned a partner, with the exception that no man was assigned to a woman who was taller than he was. Unbeknownst to the subjects, each of the partners had been coded beforehand in terms of their degree of physical attractiveness. The sole predictor of whether a subject later found his or her partner attractive (how much they liked the partner, how eager they were to date the partner again, and how often they asked the partner later for a date) was the partner's degree of physical attractiveness (which, I would argue, was in fact sexual attractiveness). Things like personality or intelligence had no predictive value.

It is significant to note here that while it was the degree of physical attractiveness that determined whether a subject found his or her partner attractive, this had little predictive value in determining whether the encounter would evolve into a long-term relationship. When the subjects were contacted six months later to see if they had dated since their first encounter, it was found that the couples who were most likely to have done so were those who had a similar degree of physical attractiveness. This supports what is known as the matching hypothesis, namely, the idea that people tend to have partners who match their own level of physical attractiveness, a view that has received support from other studies.[18] However, it only supports the matching hypothesis for long-term relationships. The other findings of the study seem to support the idea that it is physical attractiveness that initially determines whether someone finds another person attractive as a partner (not similar levels of physical attractiveness).

The question of why similarity of physical attractiveness plays a role in sexual attraction, albeit in sexual attraction that leads to long-term relationships, is one that has no definite answer. And it is important to see here that the matching hypothesis, in its most basic form, is simply a statement about the fact of matching, not what causes the matching. Various views, however, have been put forward. One view uses the idea of "level of aspiration." This account is that people who are considered unattractive simply cannot attract someone who is considered attractive. Because of their knowledge of their own unattractiveness and their fear of rejection by an attractive person, they accordingly change their level of aspiration and make do with someone whose physical attractiveness is at their own level.[19]

Although this view is no doubt true in some cases, there are problems with accepting it as a general account. One problem is that it is not clear that people are fully aware of their own level of attractiveness. It is not uncommon to find people who are quite incapable of rating their own attractiveness, people who are confident they are attractive when others do not think so, and people who are convinced that they are unattractive when in fact they are quite attractive. And even if someone does have an accurate awareness, there is also the common element of manipulation that is used in trying to attract a partner. That is, rather than resigning themselves to an unattractive partner, many people may try to manipulate an attractive partner into accepting them. A woman, for example, may be aware of her lower level of attractiveness when compared to a man to whom she is sexually attracted. Rather than simply give up, however, she might try to gain his interest by being especially affectionate to him, dressing in a way that he likes, or tantalizing him with vague offers of sex, or even actual sex.

This sort of manipulation to attract a partner who might otherwise seem unattainable is an age-old practice found in many cultures. In the *Kāma*

Sūtra, for example, Vātsyāyana, the sūtra's author, recommends the trick of pretending to be ill in order to start to gain a woman's interest: "When she comes to him, he gets her to rub his head; and he takes her hand and places it, feelingly, on his eyes and forehead. Under the pretext of preparing medicines, he charges her with something to do . . . he lets her go only after getting her to promise to return. He uses this method for three nights and three twilights."[20] This suggests that it is not so uncommon for people to attempt to attract others who are beyond their expected level of aspiration.

Another view is that since attractive people will choose other attractive people and have no trouble in obtaining them, other less attractive people are left with no alternative except to choose less attractive people. On this view it is not that, because of fear of rejection, unattractive people decide to choose other such people. Rather, there are no others left to choose from.[21] This account, however, also has difficulties. For although it might seem a possible explanation when considered from a vague theoretical level, it does not fit with what clearly goes on around us. That is, it is simply not true that whenever a person starts to look for a partner, all the people who are more attractive than him or her are already taken. It should be obvious that there are always numerous attractive people who are not taken or who were once taken but now are available. And even if they were all taken, being taken by one person in no way implies that someone cannot be taken away by someone else. It happens all the time.

Before I suggest another way to explain the phenomenon of matching in partner choice, I should first point out that although these are different variables—how attractive a person is in himself or herself versus how similar his or her physical attractiveness is to another person's—both are nevertheless still instances of physical appearance. It therefore looks like physical appearance plays a decisive role in both initial and long-term sexual attraction.

But how then does the matching hypothesis fit with the idea that, when it comes to long-term relationships, what is important is similarity of personality? This requires explanation because the matching hypothesis is a claim about the basic role of physical appearance, whereas the other is a claim about the basic role of personality. How, then, do these two distinct accounts fit together? One likely answer, it seems to me, is that while both are conditions for the persistence of a long-term relationship, similarity of level of physical attractiveness is a more basic condition than similarity of personality. Therefore, the similarity of another person's personality to one's own is only attractive if that person has a similar level of physical attractiveness. Here, too, it is physical appearance that plays the primary role in sexual attraction.

One idea that appears to stand in the way of accepting this account is that females are just not sexually attracted to physical appearance in the way that males are. And this view persists despite the finding of the just-mentioned study and others that appear to have replicated the results.[22] Female sexual attraction to physical appearance is expressed well by a woman who says that, in choosing a sexual partner, "He must be fit, in shape, not overweight. He cannot have a belly. I like nice hair. He must be clean. I want him showered and smelling good. He has to have a butt; something I can grab and there'll be some meat in my hand."[23] It also does not take too much observation to notice that, like men, women also tend to decide on someone's sexual attractiveness merely by glancing at him (or smelling him). Perhaps such a physical evaluation does not typically lead a woman to pursue or make herself available to an unknown man, but this does not negate the fact that she is still responding to what she sees as the man's sexual attractiveness. It also looks like the personality of the attractive person is, for the female, normally allowed to become an element in consideration only after the man is seen to have certain sexually attractive physical characteristics.[24] (This seems also, to some extent, true for the male's interest in a female's personality.)[25]

For example, we have all heard the phrase "tall, dark, and handsome," which is meant to express a female preference for what females typically see as a sexually attractive man. And one cannot help but notice that nothing about personality appears in the phrase, each element of which refers to a physical feature. Further, although the phrase is something of a cliché and therefore might seem to have little to do with what women actually find attractive, it cannot be so easily dismissed. This is indicated by a man's tallness—not absolute tallness, but tallness in relation to a female's height—being called the "cardinal principle of dating."[26] In other words, a major rule guiding sexual partner choice is that the man should be taller than the woman. This tendency is so strong that one American study found out that only in 1 out of 720 dating couples was the female taller than the male.[27] Although this is an American study, it would seem likely that the same cardinal principle of partner choice occurs across cultures (at least in cultures where choice is allowed). It is true that in all cultures women tend to be shorter than men, which would make it likely that a female would end up with a man who was taller than her. But more seems to be going on here than mere probability, for women tend to express a preference for men who are taller than them. One might still wonder if it is male preference for shorter women that is really responsible for men ending up with shorter women.

There is, however, evidence to suggest that while it is often important for a female that she is not taller than her male partner, men are not so bothered about the height of their female partners.[28] This, however, is just a tendency.

Coming, then, to the second element in "tall, dark, and handsome," this also might well be an element in female sexual preference. Although it is unclear what "dark" refers to (perhaps eyes, hair, or skin), it is also true that, in addition to having the tendency to be taller than women, men tend to have slightly darker-pigmented skin than women of the same ethnic group.[29] This might suggest that "dark" refers to the man's skin color in relation to the woman's skin color. This is supported by evidence suggesting that women have a somewhat greater preference for men with darker skin color, while men have a similar preference for women with a fairer skin color.[30]

As for "handsome," this, too, would seem to suggest a physical feature, here probably referring to perceived facial or overall physical appearance. It is interesting, however, that no specific quality is mentioned here. "Tall" and "dark" might not be too specific, but at least it is clear enough what the qualities refer to. "Handsome," on the other hand, might refer to many different qualities. Since it is probably meant to encompass sexually attractive facial features, the lack of specificity is understandable. For, as I shall argue, the idea of what constitutes sexually attractive facial features (as opposed to merely physically attractive) is an area where, for both men and women, there is disagreement.

All of this seems to indicate that sexual attraction operates in a way that is relatively free from the constraints imposed on other forms of interpersonal attraction. There are, however, two forms of attraction that might seem to be exceptions to this claim. One is romantic love and the other is affiliation. Romantic love seems an exception because in some cases it looks like people can fall in love in the absence of any knowledge about the beloved's personality. What I have in mind is the phenomenon of "love at first sight," as it is often called. In such a situation, one individual purportedly sees another for the first time and immediately falls in love with the person. A variation of this might be called "love at many sights." In this situation, one individual might see another individual on different occasions—all the while never meeting the person or knowing anything about his or her personality—before developing romantic feelings toward that person. Both situations are clearly distinct from the other, more common situation in which a person meets another, spends time with him or her, and, after getting to know the other person, then falls in love. In "love at first sight" or its variation, romantic attraction might seem to be free from constraints in the same way that sexual attraction is.

One could question this, however, by asking whether love at first sight really exists in the first place. And there is at least one article with the title of "The Myth of Love at First Sight." Still, there are people who report the experience of love at first sight, and everyday observation suggests it does happen, though how common it is or how long it lasts are other questions. The reason, then, why romantic attraction seems to operate in the same way as sexual attraction is that sexual attraction is an integral part of romantic attraction. That is, the reason one can become romantically attracted to someone while knowing little of the individual's personality is merely that such attraction is a result of the sexual attraction that is part of romantic love. Just how this integration occurs is something I will discuss further in Chapter Five.

It could be objected here that romantic feelings need not have anything to do with sexual attraction. When we are romantically attracted to someone, the objection could say, having sex with the person might be the farthest thing from our mind. This, it could then be concluded, shows that sexual attraction is not an integral part of romantic attraction.

By way of reply, however, one could ask, "What about sensual embracing, passionate kissing, or caressing of naked skin? Are these actions performed with the beloved also the farthest from our mind?" The idea that such warm and intimate interactions with the beloved have nothing to do with romantic attraction seems highly dubious. And if they do play an integral role in romantic attraction, then it seems that sexual attraction likewise plays an integral role. This is because the word "sexual" in the term "sexual attraction" need not refer to any specific form of sexual interaction. When many people think of the idea of having sex or sexual interaction, it seems they immediately think of sexual intercourse, that is, the act of a man's erect penis entering a woman's vagina. However, as should be obvious, this is only one form of sexual interaction. Fellatio, cunnilingus, anal intercourse, oral-anal contact, rubbing genitals together, fondling and sucking of the breasts, and masturbating or being masturbated by one's partner are also instances of sexual interaction.

But if it is accepted that oral-genital interaction is a form of sexual interaction, then it will be difficult to maintain that oral-anal or even oral-oral interaction (as in deep erotic kissing) are not forms of sexual interaction. And the same would seem true of sensual embracing and caressing of naked skin. The main reason someone might want to dismiss such activities as not being sexual, it would seem, is that they do not involve the genitals. But then, as the acts of fondling and sucking of the breasts and anallingus make clear, one can clearly have sexual interaction without using the genitals.

If it is then accepted that acts like sensuous embracing, passionate kissing, and caressing of naked skin are sexual interactions and, further, that thinking of such acts is part of the experience of romantic attraction, then it seems to follow that sexual attraction is part of romantic attraction. This then would explain why one can have romantic attraction to a stranger. For what is driving the romantic attraction in such a case is the component that is sexual attraction, and, as I have argued, sexual attraction also needs nothing more than a "first sight" to start it working. As the ancient Greek philosopher Aristotle put it, "The pleasure of the eye is the beginning of love. For no one loves if he has not first been delighted by the form of the beloved."[31] There are, naturally, other features of the attractive person that can drive romantic attraction, features that are not immediately discernible at first sight. Such features might include the person's personality, attitudes, or willingness to facilitate one's goals or needs. But then, as the possibility of love at first sight shows, these features are not essential elements in romantic attraction.

A second possible counter-example here is affiliation. For it could be argued that the nature of affiliation shows that sexual attraction's freedom of operation is not distinct after all. Here it might be asserted that affiliation, like sexual attraction, need not be based on any knowledge of the other person's personality or dispositions. People can, for example, feel an affiliation to another person simply because of his or her physical attractiveness.

However, although it might be true for some forms of affiliation, for other forms of affiliation it is obvious that they are essentially based on a knowledge of the person's personality or dispositions. As mentioned, people often seek out affiliation to another person because of that person's charismatic admired abilities. Or again, one might desire affiliation to someone who has an ability or personality trait that one enjoys. Maybe the person has a good sense of humor or musical abilities, and by being affiliated to that person, one gets to enjoy his or her humor or musical skills. There is also evidence that people with low self-esteem will tend to seek affiliation to people with high self-esteem.[32] In addition to this, people can seek to be affiliated with another person because of that person's connection to a particular social group. Someone might long to become a member of a particular exclusive club, say, a university fraternity or sorority, and so seek affiliation to a member of that club. This might be done for the purpose of somehow getting membership in the club, or it might simply be an attempt to get close to a member of the club in order to pretend to oneself, and maybe others, that one is somehow a member.

In none of these cases does the physical appearance of the other person play any part in the affiliative attraction. Further, evidence suggests that verbal affiliative behavior need not be influenced by physical attractiveness.[33] Moreover, there might well be situations in which the physical appearance plays a part, but it only does so if it is a physical *unattractiveness*. To give an example, one of my students told me that when she became overweight she noticed, much to her consternation, that other overweight women in her dorm began to seek out her company. The motive she discerned behind this affiliation was that by being seen in her company, these other women could deemphasize their own weight problems. Being seen with a thinner woman, on the other hand, would set up a contrast in which their weight problems would clearly stand out.

All of this shows that although some types of affiliation do not concern themselves with the attractive individual's personality or dispositions, other types do. That is, there is nothing in the nature of affiliation that renders it essentially free from considerations of the attractive person's personality or dispositions. This makes it distinct from sexual attraction, which is fundamentally based on physical appearance.

It is important to see, however, that none of this implies that one will act on the sexual attraction and pursue the possibility of having sex with the attracting person. Sexual attraction here refers only to the experience of feeling sexually attracted to another person, not to the behavior of definitely seeking a sexual encounter. I mention this here because a natural response might be to reject this account of sexual attraction because one feels it implies pursuing sexual contact with friends, affiliates, and strangers; in short, with anyone whom one finds sexually attractive. With this idea in mind, the objection might be, "But I could never have sexual attraction to someone whom I only want as a friend, or an affiliate or, worse, to someone whom I do not even want to be affiliated with." Such an objection, however, only gets its force if the phrase "have sexual attraction to" is taken to mean something like "sexually pursue" or "actually try to have sex with." For, of course, there are numerous factors or concerns in peoples' lives that will make them not want to act on every sexual attraction they feel. Many people will only want sex with someone they like, or only within a romantic relationship. They might be too busy, lack self-confidence, or be racked with guilt. Or perhaps they are already in a sexual relationship and, for any number of reasons, do not want a further sexual relationship. Or, more basically, they might simply be aware of the impracticability of acting on every instance of sexual attraction. Fortunately, however, the phrase "have sexual attraction to" does not mean "try to have sex with." It merely means to feel oneself sexually attracted to someone.

In addition to this, it is important to note that to find someone sexually attractive—that is, to be sexually attracted to the person—is something quite different from noticing that someone is sexually attractive from a point of view that is not one's own. Thus, a heterosexual woman can easily notice that another woman is sexually attractive from a man's point of view without herself being sexually attracted to the woman. She could, for example, notice that the other woman has various features that men would typically find sexually attractive. Yet she herself being heterosexual, does not find the other woman sexually attractive. In other words, she does not feel sexual attraction toward the woman. Therefore, to find another person sexually attractive is quite different from noting that the person has the quality of sexual attraction for people other than oneself. This is something that one can easily do without feeling sexually attracted to that person. To find a person sexually attractive is to experience that person's attraction as working on oneself. It is to enter into an intimate if nonreciprocal relationship with the other person such that one is under the sway of that person's sexual attraction.

It seems, then, that sexual attraction does operate in a way that is fundamentally different from other forms of attraction. But why is that? Why is it that sexual attraction need not concern itself with the attractive person's personality, attitudes, or other such psychological characteristics? The obvious answer is that sexual attraction focuses primarily on the physical features of the attracter. This would seem to suggest that sexual attraction is basically physical attraction. And a look at the literature in this area will show that most, if not all, researchers dealing with sexual attraction draw no distinction between it and physical attraction. They simply refer to the former as if it were the same thing as the latter.

However, a little reflection makes it plain that, even though related, the two cannot be the same thing. For one thing, someone can agree that a person of the desired gender is physically attractive but nevertheless feel that he or she "is not my type" or "does not do it for me." That is, he or she does not find the person sexually attractive. For another thing, heterosexuals can find members of their own sex physically attractive and yet, because they are heterosexual, not find them sexually attractive. Similarly, homosexuals can easily experience members of the opposite sex as being physically attractive and, because they are homosexuals, not find them sexually attractive.

Further, homosexual and heterosexual males disagree on what sort of male faces are attractive, with homosexual males preferring more masculine male faces and heterosexuals preferring more feminine male faces. Also, homosexual and heterosexual males disagree on what sort of female faces are attractive, with homosexual males preferring more masculine female faces and heterosexuals preferring more feminine female faces.[34] Similarly, lesbians and heterosexual females disagreed on what sort of female faces are more attractive. Here lesbians preferred slightly more masculine female faces, while heterosexual women preferred feminine female faces. The reason for this, I would suggest, is that homosexual men and women consider same-sex faces more in terms of sexual attraction, while heterosexuals consider them in terms of nonsexual physical attraction.

The reverse of this is also true, namely, that people can find someone sexually attractive while not finding him or her to be physically attractive. A man, for example, might find a woman of a particular build, perhaps having disproportionately large buttocks, to be highly sexually attractive and yet not find such a feature to be physically attractive. That is, when considering her from a nonsexual point of view, he does not find her to be aesthetically pleasing. Supporting this view is the fact that there are several erotic publications that portray individuals whom most people would probably see as physically unattractive in sexual positions or engaged in sexual acts. These images are made available for the obvious reason that there are people who find such individuals to be sexually attractive. There is also the phenomenon of people being sexually attracted to persons with deformities or amputations, features that might otherwise be considered physically unattractive.[35] One might be tempted to think here that if someone finds an individual sexually attractive, then he or she must also find the person physically attractive, even if others do not. But I have not seen any evidence for this claim. Indeed, it might even be that it is the model's physical unattractiveness that renders him or her sexually attractive for some people.

Furthermore, it is noteworthy that nonhuman objects that are experienced as having sexual attraction are not also described as physically attractive. What I have in mind here are cases of fetishism wherein an individual finds nonhuman objects to be sexually attractive. That is, it seems that individuals with a fetish for clothing, shoes, or handbags will experience these objects as having sexual attraction in the same sense in which other people experience a person as having sexual attraction. They will not, however, experience them as being physically attractive in the same way that people experience human beings as being physically attractive. For physical attraction is a quality that seems tied to the idea of facial or overall human appearance.

Although this is also true for sexual attraction, the power of sexual attraction seems to be able to transfer itself more easily to mere symbols of the body or to things merely associated with the body.

Finally, evidence suggests that people typically regarded as physically attractive often receive preferential treatment and better evaluations from both members of their own sex and the opposite sex[36] and that physical attraction plays a role in the formation of friendships and other relationships that have little to do with sexual attraction.[37] All of this indicates that sexual attraction, though tied to physical attraction, is something more than mere physical attraction. This is not to say that there will be no gray areas between the two, areas where it will be unclear whether it is physical or sexual attraction that one is feeling. One might, for example, see someone as being only physically attractive and then at some point gradually become aware that one now sees that person as being sexually attractive. Yet just where one's experience changed from physical to sexual attraction may be unclear.

ALLURE

But what is this something more that essentially distinguishes sexual from physical attraction? To answer this, it must first be seen that sexual attraction itself has various interrelated components, such as the social, behavioral, biological, and experiential components. In studying the phenomenon of sexual attraction, one can, for example, examine the social structures in which sexual attraction occurs or the cohesive or disruptive roles that sexual attraction plays within various social units. One could also examine the behaviors associated with sexual attraction, say, gaze, proximity, or touching. Or the main point of focus could be the biological events that might occur in sexual attraction: increased heart rate, increased perspiration, changes in the genitals, and so on. Finally, one could investigate the experiential aspect of sexual attraction, namely, the way in which sexual attraction presents itself to our awareness.

Now, although each of these components plays a role in the wider phenomenon of sexual attraction, it is in the experiential element that sexual attraction takes on the crucial meaning it has in our lives. For it is within our experience that sexual attraction grabs hold of us and announces itself as something that cannot be ignored. And this is true whether we act on our sexual attraction or not. It is in experience that we undergo its unique and compelling character, a character that singles out another person by directing our awareness to a peculiar effect that the person has on us. This is the effect of making us sexually attracted to the other person. It is in this way that the experiential component constitutes the meaningful core of sexual attraction. This does not imply that the social, behavioral, or biological elements are not important but only emphasizes that it is the experiential component that is crucial for giving sexual attraction the importance it has for us. The social, behavioral, and biological elements are variable and so are not definitive of the essence of sexual attraction. The experience, however, constitutes the heart of sexual attraction, and were it to be removed, whatever was left would not be sexual attraction as we know it.

With this much made clear, I should like to suggest that what essentially distinguishes sexual attraction from physical attraction is the experience of something that can be called "allure." Allure is what a person who is perceived to be sexually attractive emanates toward those who come under the sway of his or her sexual attraction. As a noun, the word "allure" carries meanings like "attractiveness," "charm," "enticement," and "fascination." In its verbal form, it means "to tempt," "to entice," or "to charm." However, none of these meanings of allure need convey the idea of sexual attraction. One reason is that we can also be attracted to, charmed by, or enticed by nonsexual things, places, or lifestyles. With this idea in mind, we can easily refer to the allure of the Orient, the allure of a pirate's life, or some such thing, with no idea of sexual attraction implied.

Another reason is that people can also present an allure to others where the allure is not overtly related to the physical features of the person. This seems to be the case with the allure of charismatic persons or of those who might be intensely admired for their abilities or achievements. In these sorts of situations the allure someone feels need not involve sexual attraction. Nevertheless, it seems significant that here, too, where the allure is given off by a person, sexual attraction might still play a role in the allure.

A good example of this is seen in the film *American Beauty*. Here, real estate agent Carolyn, who is having much difficulty selling houses, becomes deeply envious of Buddy, a competing real estate agent who does remarkably well selling houses. She becomes full of admiration and is awe-struck by his ability, plainly finding him alluring. The allure he has for her, however, leads her to experience a sexual attraction to him and finally to having sexual intercourse with him.

It is important to note, however, that even though the allure in this situation seems primarily related to a person's ability rather than his physical appearance, Carolyn is nevertheless very aware of his physical appearance. This is because Buddy has posted (as real estate agents are keen to do) larger-than-life pictures of himself on billboard advertisements throughout the town. As a result, Carolyn is, wherever she goes, continually haunted by his image. This would suggest that in the allure she feels for Buddy—an allure in which sexual attraction is not fully absent—physical appearance might still be involved.

But, one could ask, if sexual attraction is operating in this instance of allure, is this not only because the persons in question are male and female and both heterosexual? What about the case in which the person experiencing the allure and the alluring individual are both of the same sex and both heterosexual? Clearly a heterosexual person can be allured in this way by someone of the same sex and so not experience the allure in a necessarily sexual way. We could, for instance, imagine a variation of the story of *American Beauty*. Here it might be an apparently heterosexual male who becomes awestruck by and envious of Buddy. In such a situation we could imagine that the man feels an allure toward Buddy, yet feels no sexual attraction.

My reply is yes, I agree that we could imagine this situation. Nevertheless, even here it might well be difficult to distinguish an allure involving sexual attraction from a nonsexual allure. This is because homosexuality is not an all-or-nothing affair. Some people who describe themselves as "heterosexual" can still experience homosexual attractions.[38] This would seem especially so when the allure to a same-sexed person is at least partially based on physical appearance. If a man were to find another man alluring because of his physical appearance, most people would probably see this as being a case of homosexual attraction or at least an attraction with homosexual elements.

It seems, therefore, that there is an ordinary sense of "allure" that, particularly when based on physical appearance, means "sexual attraction" or "sexual attractiveness." This is the sense that is used in, for example, the journal article entitled "The universal allure of the hourglass figure."[39] It is also the sense that is used in the title of the popular women's magazine *Allure*, where all the accessories of female sexual attraction—makeup, clothing, hairstyles, for example—along with how to get an hourglass figure, are discussed and illustrated in detail.

This idea of allure also helps to draw another important distinction. This is the distinction between sexual attraction and sexual desire, a distinction most researchers have failed to notice. Consequently, many people end up using these two terms interchangeably as if they were the same thing. Once it is seen, however, that sexual attraction encompasses the idea of allure but sexual desire does not, then the distinction between the two ideas is a bit easier to understand. The reason they do not denote the same thing is that allure is experienced as coming from the person one is sexually attracted to. That is, it is the sexually attractive person who is experienced as having allure. Sexual desire, on the other hand is not something the desired person has, it is something the *desiring* person has. That is, someone who experiences sexual desire for another person experiences it as an urge from within that is directed outward to the desired person.[40] This is quite distinct from the experience of being allured by another person.

But then what is it about this sense of allure that enables sexual attraction to be distinguished from mere physical attraction? The answer, I should like to argue, is found in three interrelated features of the experience of allure, features that are not present in the experience of mere physical attraction. These are the features of feeling oneself being drawn toward the attractive person, a sense of helplessness in being thus drawn, and sexual fantasies about the result of being drawn.

The first feature refers to the characteristic sensation of having oneself pulled toward the person who emanates the sexual attraction. This does not mean that one is actually pulled across space toward the individual who is attractive, but only that there is a distinct sensation in one's awareness of being drawn toward the person. In such cases the drawing toward takes on a near magnetic quality: one experiences a persistent tug toward the sexually attractive person in much the same way that a nail—if it could experience things—might feel the pull of a nearby magnet.

This is not to say that the sensation need be overwhelming. It can, but there are degrees of this attraction. At one end of the spectrum the subtle attractions from the person are barely felt. Here they are merely a faint reminder that the other person's features have a hold on one's awareness, pulling at one's attention, as it were. It is because of such weak sensations that it might in some cases be difficult to discern where mere physical attraction ends and sexual attraction begins. At the other end, one seems to be "swept off one's feet"—as the telling expression goes—and powerfully drawn to the attractive person. In this case one feels swept off one's feet by the attracting person, much like a nail is swept off the table by a powerful magnet. In all cases, however, there persists the sensation of feeling oneself being drawn to the other person. Moreover, this sensation of being drawn is one that occurs in the diverse instances of sexual attraction. It is the magnetic pull that makes it difficult for people to look away from sexually attractive opposite-sex faces, and it is the forceful pull that draws one toward the naked body of one's partner in the moment before an embrace.[41] Finally, the presence of the sexually attractive person not only creates the sensation of being pulled toward him or her, but he or she also seems to pull forth ideas, images, and imaginings from the attracted individual. These are mental representations of the intimate physical joining, which present themselves as the goal of the pulling.

The second feature of allure—that of a sense of helplessness—is interwoven with the first. This is because the sensation of being drawn toward the attractive person carries with it a sense of being drawn helplessly. In the moment one sees the other person as sexually attractive, one feels drawn beyond one's will. This is because the pull of the other person is something that one senses as coming from the other person, not from oneself, just as the pull of the magnet comes from the magnet, not the nail. Consequently, it gives the sensation of being beyond one's control. This does not mean that in experiencing the sexual attraction of another person one loses all control or has no free will in deciding how one will act toward the attractive person. It only means that the attraction seems to work of its own accord, having little to do with one's own effort. It might even work against one's effort. Therefore, although I may try to disengage my awareness of the attractive person by looking elsewhere or thinking about something else, I nevertheless feel her attraction dismantling these attempts, pushing them aside, and drawing my gaze and thoughts back to her.

This should not be taken to imply that one cannot help being sexually attracted but only that if one does feel sexual attraction, then it will more or less contain the element of helplessness. (It is again because of the "less" possibility that there might appear gray areas where the distinction between physical and sexual attraction is not clearly discerned.) One can, of course, work against this sensation of loss of control and even overcome it. But if one overcomes it completely, then what one experiences will no longer be sexual attraction. This is because the experience of sexual attraction is, in its essence, the experience of helplessness before the attracting qualities of the sexually attractive person.

The third feature of allure is the presence of sexual fantasies that center around the result of being drawn to the attractive person. This feature is also interwoven with the other two. I just mentioned that the feature of being drawn involves the provoking of ideas, images, and imaginings of an intimate physical joining with the attractive person. These thoughts are none other than sexual fantasies of oneself in a sexual encounter with the attractive person.

Some people might feel that they could only have sexual fantasies about their sexual or romantic partners and not about any sexually attractive person they see. One survey even found that 48 percent of those asked felt it was not "OK" to have sexual fantasies about a nonpartner.[42] Although the most usual sexual fantasy seems to involve imagining having sexual intercourse with one's past or current partner, evidence suggests that fantasies about nonpartners are quite common and, further, that there is little difference between men and women in this regard. One study, for example, found that in the two months before the study, 98 percent of men and 80 percent of women had sexual fantasies about someone who was not their current partner. This was true regardless of the subject's marital status.[43]

But who are these other people who become the subjects of our sexual fantasies? They are, I would argue, those we find sexually attractive. Further, although such fantasies can occur in the absence of the sexually attractive person, they also occur in the moment we decide he or she is sexually attractive. For to find someone sexually attractive is just to experience oneself as being attracted or pulled toward the person for the purpose of a sexual encounter. This shows a striking feature of the experience of sexual attraction. It is not just that one experiences the other person. Rather one experiences an idea, image, or imagining of the other person brought together with a similar representation of oneself. That is, the allure of the other person fundamentally involves representations of oneself. In experiencing the attractive person's allure, the attracted person can immediately discern herself. This is what the presence of the sexual fantasies shows.

Again, it must be remembered that sexual encounters can be of numerous kinds and do not refer just to sexual intercourse or even genital contact. Naked fondling, caressing, and erotic kissing are also forms of sexual encounters and, accordingly, sexual fantasies can also encompass these sorts of sexual activities. Further, they can focus on different people in different ways. They can focus on one or more specific persons, or they can be on no one in particular, say, nameless or faceless persons who are unknown to the fantasizer. In taking a person for its object, a sexual fantasy can conjure up representations of a solitary person, someone who is, say, undressing, bathing, or masturbating. Or they can take as their object imaginings of two or more people who are intimately joined through sexually interaction. Or instead of involving persons, they can involve specific parts of the person's body or things that symbolize the body. Moreover, sexual fantasies can take place during a sexual encounter, in order to increase sexual interest or desire or facilitate sexual pleasure or orgasm during the encounter. Or they might occur when one is alone with one's thoughts or during masturbation. In addition, sexual fantasies can be scripted or unscripted. That is, they can follow a fixed story line or format, or they can be more spontaneous, developing in more make-it-up-as-you-go-along sort of way.[44] It is also significant that people tend mainly to fantasize about current or past sexual partners and specific sexual interactions with them, especially those interactions that are found to be particularly arousing. As Peter Doskoch puts it in his discussion of sexual fantasies, "Despite the potential for limitless freedom, our fantasies generally stay firmly tethered to reality."[45]

There are also various gender differences in sexual fantasies. The main one seems to be that while men tend to imagine doing something to a woman while focusing on her body, a woman tends to imagine a man doing something to her while focusing on his desire for her.[46] These are but a few of the forms that sexual fantasies can take.

The sexual fantasies that take place in allure, however, are of a particular kind. Unfortunately, however, very little research has been done on these instances of sexual fantasy. From my discussions with students and others, however, I have come to see that in the experience of allure, these fantasies specifically involve ideas, images, or imaginings of the fantasizer's own body intimately joined with the body of the sexually attractive person whom one is in the process of observing. Further, although many sexual fantasies can involve extended developments and story lines, the fantasies of allure will tend to be brief and immediate. Although other sexual fantasies can be brief and fleeting, those that are part of allure are distinguished by their being provoked by the observation or idea of a sexually attractive individual.

The idea of being provoked is an important one, for sexual fantasies are often imaginings that a person actively engages in. In such fantasies one has the sense of choosing the fantasy and directing it by oneself. In the brief fantasies of allure, however, the fantasies can have a spontaneous quality where they are provoked or brought forth not by any choosing on one's own part, but rather by the awareness of the sexually attractive person. It is this self-generated quality that ties such fantasies to the other two features of allure, namely, the sensation of being drawn toward the other person and the sense of helplessness in being thus drawn. For if the sexual images are provoked by my perception of the other person, and if these images attract me, then there is a sense in which they are working to draw me toward the other person. Also, if they present themselves as appearing beyond my active choosing, then there is a sense in which I am helpless before them. They seem to just appear of their own accord. They are, to use a technical term in psychology, autochthonic and therefore appear not be under the person's control. Also, the brevity of the fantasies of allure will tend to distinguish them from other more extended fantasies that might occur in an extended encounter with a particular person. The brevity of these fantasies might even, in some instances, cause someone to overlook or not clearly notice the fantasy. However, listening to descriptions of the experience of sexual attraction has convinced me that some sort of fantasy image is normally present.

The fantasy here is the end result of the sensation of being drawn to the attractive person. The fantasized image is invoked by the very sensation of being pulled toward the other person. For in being pulled toward the other person, one cannot help but see the end result to which the sensation of being pulled is leading one, namely, an intimate joining with the attractive person's body. If one were to let oneself go, letting the sensation of being drawn take over, then one would be taken straight into an intimate physical merging with the other person. It is this end result of the pulling that materializes in the attracted person's awareness as a sexual fantasy, albeit a brief and immediate fantasy.

One could, of course, spin such a fantasy out, extending it into various other events and story lines. But in being thus extended, it loses its immediate connection to the experience of allure. The reason for this is that if I start developing a fantasy about the person who is before me, then I have lost my immediate connection of sexual attraction to her. I am no longer in the grip of her attraction but am rather involved in the unfolding of a fantasy. This removes my awareness from the other elements of the attractive person's allure, namely, my being drawn toward her and the sense of helplessness in being drawn toward her.

This, then, is the structure of the experiential phenomenon of sexual attraction, and it is in this sense that I will be using the words "allure" and its cognates. When I use the term "sexual attraction," I will be referring to the wider phenomenon of sexual attraction. Even the term "experience of sexual attraction" does not have precisely the same meaning as "allure." This is because "the experience of sexual attraction" could also encompass the experience of the social, behavioral, and biological aspects of sexual attraction. The wider phenomena of sexual attraction and experience of sexual attraction include allure but are not limited to it.

With this much in place, it now becomes clear how sexual attraction differs fundamentally from physical attraction. Thus, the reason why the attraction I feel to the woman in the airport lounge is sexual attraction is the allure she emanates toward me. It is not simply that I note that she is good-looking or has aesthetically pleasing physical features and that is the end of it. It is rather that she allures me toward her: in the same instant that I see her as sexually attractive, I feel myself drawn helplessly in her direction. In feeling myself thus drawn, I am immediately brought to the imagining of my body intimately joining with hers. I feel her alluring me to mold my lips into hers, run my fingers through her hair and down her neck, and press my thighs up against hers, while taking her hand in mine, and so on. This is my sexual fantasy about her and me intimately joined.

These imaginings of taking her in my arms and merging with her are the mental representations of what I feel her sexual attractiveness is pulling me toward. They are elements in the instantaneous sexual fantasy that presents itself to my awareness in the moment of allure. It is, however, important to recall here that none of this need be intended by the woman. Indeed, in this case she is not even aware that I am noticing her: she is merely sitting quietly reading her book. The allure that she emanates toward me is simply her sexually attractive physical appearance operating on me.

These features of experiencing oneself being drawn beyond one's will to a close physical merging with another person's body—which are captured in the idea of allure—are absent in mere physical attraction. As I mentioned, if somebody finds another person physically attractive, he or she will tend to treat that person in a preferential way. Nothing in such treatment, however, implies that the attracted person feels himself or herself being nearly helplessly drawn into a physical intimacy, which appears in fantasy, with the physically attractive person. In other words, the merely physically attractive person has no allure for those who find him or her to be only physically attractive.

Allure also works to distinguish sexual attraction from physical attraction in another way. This is because, although people can often agree on what features count as physically attractive, what is experienced as sexually attractive seems a far more personal affair and frequently the basis of disagreement. Anyone who has discussed this topic with others will know that people can strongly disagree about what counts as a sexually attractive individual. Thus, for example, although a woman might well agree with other women that a particular man is physically attractive—that he fits the various criteria for a physically attractive man—she might nevertheless feel that he "just doesn't do it" for her. She might even understand why other women might find him sexually attractive—he could, after all, be tall dark, and handsome. However, as far as her own experience goes, she does not find this enough to make him sexually attractive for her. What is missing is that while observing him she does not feel herself being drawn helplessly toward a physically intimate joining with him. In other words, he has no allure for her.

THE ORIGINS OF ALLURE

But how could this be? How is it that a heterosexual person could see an individual of the opposite sex as physically attractive and yet not feel allured to him or her? This is a complicated issue, and no doubt there are numerous factors that can play various roles here: the observer's personality, self-esteem, and earlier sexual relationships are all possible candidates. With women, it seems that attraction to more masculine-like features in men's faces is expressed during the ovulation phase of the menstrual cycle.[47] Although this fact might be cited as accounting for why women can disagree on which men they find attractive, or at least sexually attractive, I am not sure how this could play much of a role. My suspicion would be that women at the same point in their menstrual cycle would still not agree on the exact same man as being the most sexually attractive. Even here, I would surmise, one particular man's physical appearance might just not "do it" for one woman, even though he might be seen as highly sexually attractive by another. Moreover, it is exceedingly unclear how these hormonal findings could help to explain the matching hypothesis (I will come back to these findings later).

There is, however, one possible causal explanation that seems especially prominent here. This explanation can be found in the early years of the individual's sexual development. According to Sigmund Freud, the psychologist who first explored childhood sexuality, the template for the experience of sexual attraction—the core of which is allure—is formed in the Oedipal complex.[48] This is an episode in early childhood in which the child develops strong erotic attachments to the opposite-sex parent. (Here is one place where kinship becomes interpersonal attraction.) For both the infant boy and girl the first such attachment is to the primary caregiver, which is typically the mother. For the little girl, however, these feelings are soon transferred to the father. Freud places the beginning of this transference to the father somewhere between the fifth and sixth year of age. My observations, however, suggest that it can, depending on the involvement of the father, start much earlier, perhaps already in the first year. As with the mother, it is not important that the male figure is the biological or even adoptive father, but only that he is someone who plays the role of a father, perhaps an older brother, uncle, or close man friend of the mother (I shall discuss this transference of the girl's feelings to the father more fully in the next chapter.)

In this way, then, the opposite-sex parent becomes an early object of sexual attraction for the child. These are among the first sexual feelings that are directed at another person. They are impulses that occur naturally in response to the warmth and comfort of being held, cuddled, caressed, and tended to. Because of the infant's lack of communication skills (compared to the adult's) and because of its small size and its need for physical care, much of the interaction with the caregiver is in the form of physical touching: being picked up and cradled, being cuddled, fed, cleaned, and kept warm. These early physical interactions, which are deeply enjoyed by the infant, are the blueprint for later sexual interactions and feelings.

A basic task for the developing child is then to transfer these feelings from the opposite-sex parent to another opposite-sex person outside the family and thus to experience sexual attraction to someone else. Because, however, such impulses were formed in relation to the parent, traces of the contents of these early childhood impulses remain when they are transferred later in life to potential sexual partners. Among these traces are sexually attractive images of the opposite-sex parent. As a result, people tend to be sexually attracted to those who in some way resemble their opposite-sex parent.

Although the support for this view originally comes from psychoanalytic investigations,[49] there is other evidence that points in this direction. In one study, for example, women were asked to rank various images of male physiques on a scale starting from those that looked most like their father to those that looked least like their father. They were later asked to choose the physique that they would most like in an ideal lover. The results were that the women showed a significant tendency to choose the physiques that most looked like their father or those that least looked like their father. This indicates that the women's image of their father's body played an important role (either positive or negative) in their idea of what was sexually attractive.[50] Similarly, research indicates that women who have had highly positive relationships with their father will see as attractive those male faces that have proportions similar to their father's face.[51] And this does not seem only true for biologically related daughters and fathers. The husbands of adoptive daughters also show a facial resemblance to the daughter's father.[52]

The same is true of males and their choice of sexual partners. One study showed that judges were able to match photographs of wives with photographs of the wives' mothers-in-law at a rate that was significantly higher than chance. It was also shown that the similarity in appearance between the wife and her mother-in-law was significantly higher than the similarity between the wife and her husband.[53] This indicates that men tend to choose women who resemble their mothers.

It is interesting to note that just as different women tend to prefer different male physiques, different men tend to prefer different female physiques. Although it has been frequently argued that the male preference for the hourglass figure is universal, this claim seems limited in various ways. First, there is evidence to suggest that what is thought of as the ideal female figure has changed in different historical periods. For example, one of the earliest representations of the female figure is found in a statuette known as the Venus or Woman of Willendorf. This miniature carving, which is about 27,000 years old, depicts a woman with not only excessively large breasts and buttocks, but also a protrusive midriff (the fact that it is the midriff rather than just the belly that protrudes indicates that her extra weight is not meant to be due to pregnancy). Although it is difficult to say what the motive was in making this figurine, the prominent breasts and buttocks suggest a sexual motive. It does not seem unreasonable to suppose that the culture in which this artwork was made, found the figurine's proportions—which are nothing like an hourglass—to be sexually attractive. Similar things could be said about the naked women in paintings by renaissance masters like Titian and Peter Paul Rubens. In many of these works, the women have small breasts and are fairly plump through the waist and hips, displaying more pear-shaped than hourglass figures (See, for example, Rubens' *Venus, Cupid, Bacchus, and Ceres*). Further, in one study it was shown how the waist-to-hip ratio of Playboy centerfold models and Miss America pageant winners has varied systematically throughout the 20th century.[54] If these data can be taken as an indication of male preferences, then it seems that male preferences for women's figures can vary over time.

It is also important to be aware that a woman's figure does not occur in isolation from other aspects of her body. As a result, hourglass figures will always appear in relation to different shapes and sizes of other aspects of the woman's body. This will affect her sexual attractiveness in different ways for different men. It is well known, for example, that different men focus on different parts of a woman's body in evaluating her overall sexual attractiveness. In one study it was shown that while some men focus on a woman's breasts, others focus on the buttocks, others focus on the legs, and yet others focus on the overall size of the figure.[55] In this study men were shown silhouettes of naked females and asked to choose which they found most sexually attractive. These silhouettes varied according to whether their breasts, buttocks, thighs, or overall figures were large or small. The results were that male subjects fell into eight different groups: one group who preferred large breasts, one who preferred small breasts, one who preferred large buttocks, one who preferred small buttocks, one who preferred large thighs, one who preferred small thighs, one who preferred a large overall figure, an one who preferred a small overall figure.

Unfortunately, the researchers did not collect any data concerning the physical appearance of the mothers of these men. This is unfortunate because it would have been enlightening to see if there were any correlations between the subjects' sexual preferences and the physical appearance of their mothers. Might it be, for example, that subjects whose mothers had large breasts also tended to have a sexual preference for the female silhouettes with large breasts? Or at least that those who had a positive relationship with their mothers tended to have a sexual preference for women with similar breast, buttock, thigh, or overall bodily proportions? This would seem likely when one considers the other evidence for the maternal origins of other male sexual preferences. Although the researchers did not attempt to answer these questions, they did collect data concerning various personality features of the men in the study. This enabled them to discover correlations between various personality traits and sexual preferences. Thus, for example, men who preferred large breasts tended to be sports-minded and frequent daters, whereas men who preferred small breasts tended to be religious and submissive. Because the personality traits were the only other data collected, this makes it look like there might be a causal relation between the two. It might, for example, look like being a frequent dater causes a man to prefer large breasts or maybe the reverse: a preference for large breasts causes a man to be frequent dater. But it could be that such a causal relation does not exist, for it might be that they are effects of a common cause. It could be, for example, that having a mother with large breasts causes a man both to prefer women with large breasts and to be a frequent dater. Although there are no data available that would enable us to decide one way or the other, such an explanation sits well with other data on the Oedipal origins of male sexual preferences.

Concerning both men and women, another study found that the subjects' partners tended to have eye and hair color similar to that of their opposite-sex parents but not to their same-sex parents.[56] There is also evidence that the opposite-sex parent's personality, or at least perceived personality, will play a role in what personality characteristics are seen as attractive in a partner.[57] Although this evidence concerns personality and thus does not directly affect what is seen to be sexually attractive, it nevertheless supports the general account of the role of the opposite-sex parent in influencing sexual partner choice. Further, it seems possible that it is not just opposite-sex parents who play a role in forming an individual's sense of who is sexually attractive. Other persons in one's childhood could also wield such influence. Examples might include opposite-sex significant others such as siblings, child minders, or nursery school teachers. If a child spends much time with such an opposite-sex person, developing positive feelings toward or a strong attachment to him or her, it is understandable that the child might later experience sexual attraction to similar-looking individuals.

In this way it is easy to understand how a woman might agree that a man is physically attractive but nevertheless not find him sexually attractive. For in such an instance, the woman might be one of the many women who are sexually attracted to men who resemble their fathers. And, further, the physically attractive man she is observing might bear no resemblance to her father. And the same, to be sure, could be said of a man who finds a woman sexually attractive. For if he is one of the many men who tend to feel sexual attraction to women who resemble their mothers, and since it is not at all necessary that a physically attractive woman resemble his mother, then he could easily observe a physically attractive woman and yet not find her sexually attractive.

In all of this it is important to note that someone need not be fully conscious of the parental basis of his or her sexual attraction. That is, someone who is sexually attracted to persons resembling his or her opposite-sex parent need not be fully aware that such a resemblance is driving his or her attraction. Indeed, many such people might attempt explicitly to deny to themselves that their sexual attraction has anything to do with their opposite-sex parent, or even find the idea repulsive. In Freud's theory, however, many socially unacceptable impulses—like sexual attraction to one's own parent—take place unconsciously. This is because such impulses can lead to feelings of guilt, shame, and self-loathing. Accordingly, to defend himself or herself against such noxious feelings, the individual represses such impulses into an unconscious level of awareness. This does not mean they go away or no longer play a role in the person's psychological life, but only that the individual is not fully aware of the role they play. The reason I say "not *fully* aware" rather than simply "not aware" is that even though an impulse or idea might be unconscious, it is not, I would argue, fully cut off from awareness. That is, it exists in awareness in a disguised form, lurking on the fringes of consciousness, systematically shifting its position to avoid coming into sharp focus.

This Oedipal account of the development of sexual attraction is also supported in a roundabout way by research on similarity and sexual attraction. There is evidence, for example, that couples tend to resemble each other facially.[58] But why should one be attracted to a partner who resembles oneself? Various explanations have been given. Psychologists taking an evolutionary view try to argue that this has something to do with "optimal breeding" and the fact that some genetic similarity of mating pairs leads to a better genetic constitution in the offspring. However, the same people who say this are wont to point out the undesirable effects that inbreeding can have, using this to explain why people tend to prefer similarity more in same-sex rather than opposite-sex persons.[59] But this seems more like an attempt to have it both ways than an explanation: people prefer similar-looking partners to maximize optimal breeding and people avoid similar-looking partners to maximize optimal breeding (that is, to avoid undesirable breeding). I cannot see how this is explains anything.

Another explanation is what has been called "implicit egotism."[60] According to this view, because of implicit positive self-evaluations, we all tend to gravitate toward persons, places, and things that remind us of ourselves. Consequently, people are attracted to sexual partners who remind them of themselves, that is, have a similar appearance to themselves. But if this is true, then why do women prefer men who are taller than they are, why do men prefer women with feminine voices, and why do the majority of women and men prefer opposite-sex sex partners? These are clearly not similarities. If it were true that, in sexual attraction, we gravitate toward those who remind us of ourselves, then obviously the majority of people should be homosexual. But the majority of people are not homosexual. Therefore, similarity cannot be what evokes sexual attraction.

One could try to argue here that similarity only counts to the degree that it does not abolish the biological sex characteristics that distinguish males from females. But why should that be the case? If similarity of physical appearance really is what drives sexual attraction, then why should it not include a similarity of biological sex characteristics? Why should the majority of people not also be sexually attracted to similarity of genitals (that is, toward the same sex)? And even if some argument could be given to show why similarity loses its attraction power when it comes to the genitals (and height and bodily shape differences between males and females), one could still raise the question of why men do not typically prefer women with distinctly male facial features (not just masculine-like women's faces, but faces that actually look like men's faces) and who talk and walk like men? And why do not women typically prefer men with distinctly female facial features (not just feminine-like men's faces, but faces that actually look like female faces) and who walk and talk like women? If similarity of appearance plays an important role in sexual attraction, then again it would seem that men should be sexually attracted to women who distinctly resemble men, and women should be sexually attracted to men who distinctly resemble women. Research shows, however, that heterosexual men and women are sexually attracted to distinctly opposite-sex features in each other (though this may be less so for women than for men).[61] So, again, it does not look like similarity of appearance plays much of a role in sexual attraction.

How, then, can the similarity of appearance in sexual partners be explained? One possible explanation is that since people tend to resemble their parents (even opposite-sex parents), and since one's partner will tend to resemble oneself, then one's partner will tend to resemble one's opposite-sex parent. If we put this together with the fact that people tend to be sexually attracted to persons who resemble their opposite-sex parent, then, it is understandable that people will tend to be sexually attracted to individuals who resemble themselves. On this view, what one is sexually attracted to in someone is not the fact that he or she resembles oneself, but that he or she resembles one's opposite-sex parent. The other person's resemblance to oneself is merely a side effect of this.

This could also be an explanation for the matching hypothesis mentioned earlier. On this view, it will be recalled, people tend to have partners that reflect their own level of physical attractiveness. However, a person's level of physical attractiveness probably reflects her parents' level of physical attractiveness. It might well be, therefore, that what she is sexually attracted to in another is not that the other person has her own level of physical attractiveness but rather that the person has her own opposite-sex parent's level of physical attractiveness.

One possible way to test this explanation would be to examine the degree to which partners of adoptive children resemble the adoptive children's opposite-sex parents. This would be interesting because people who are adopted tend not to resemble their opposite-sex parent. They are, after all, adopted and so have no family resemblances with their parents. Consequently, if the partners of adoptive persons tended to resemble the adoptive persons, this could only be because adoptive persons are attracted to people who resemble themselves, not because they are attracted primarily to persons who resemble their opposite-sex parents. Although such a study remains to be done, we do know, as already stated, that the husbands of adoptive daughters do tend to resemble the adoptive daughter's opposite-sex parent. This would suggest that resemblances to the opposite-sex parent would primarily influence an adoptive person's partner choice, not resemblances to the adoptive person himself or herself.

However, even if the results of such a study indicated that it was resemblances to the person himself or herself, things are not so simple. This is because an adoptive person might well be influenced by imaginings about what his or her opposite-sex biological parent looked like. I knew, for example, an individual who was adopted and had no resemblance at all to his adoptive mother. One of the physical features that he had was prominent freckles. It also turned out that he had several girlfriends, one after the other, all of whom had prominent freckles. With only this information at hand, one might be led to conclude that he was sexually attracted to women who resembled himself. The problem with this conclusion, however, is that he also wondered much about what his biological mother must have looked like. One of the ideas that he came up with was that, like himself, she must have also had prominent freckles. Because of this, it could easily be that what attracted him to his freckled girlfriends was not that they resembled himself, but rather that they resembled his fantasized biological mother. Complexities like this show the difficulties that would surround the interpretation of the results of the study.

One question that arises out of this discussion is the question of the origin of physical attraction. Clearly, a person's criteria for physical attractiveness cannot be learned in the same way as that for sexual attractiveness, for otherwise there would be no distinction between the two. Whoever one saw as physically attractive (as long as he or she was of the appropriate gender), one would also see as sexually attractive. And, conversely, whoever one saw as sexually attractive one would also see as physically attractive. But this, as I have shown, is far from the case. Where, then, do our ideas about physical attraction come from? One idea that is currently popular is that human beings have been, through millions of years of evolution, genetically programmed to find particular features physically attractive. The purported reason for this is that these features are indicative of "good genes" and thus that the person with such features has a likelihood of producing genetically superior and viable offspring.

The first thing to notice about such an account is that it does not clearly distinguish between physical and sexual attraction. For although this might appear to explain sexual attraction, which can lead to sexual reproduction, it does not explain nonsexual physical attraction, which does not lead to reproduction. How, for example, is one man's nonsexual physical attraction (or even sexual attraction) to another man to be accounted for in terms of the attractive man's "good genes"? Since such an attraction will never lead to offspring, it could never be selected for, not at least in the same way that sexual attraction to such features might be selected for. Further, the "good gene" account does not even clearly explain sexual attraction. For, as I have argued, people tend to be sexually attracted to those who resemble their opposite-sex parent (some of whom might well have bad genes). And if the theory cannot even explain sexual attraction, then it seems unlikely that it could explain physical attraction.

An argument that is brought in here to show the evolutionary basis of people's attraction to certain physical features is the fact that infants from as young as 14–151 hours of age show a preference for gazing at attractive faces.[62] Because an infant of this age supposedly has not been influenced by cultural ideas of physical attractiveness, this, some have argued, shows that such ideas must be innate.[63]

There are, however, problems with this argument. First, just because an infant displays a particular behavior, it does not follow that when an older person displays the same behavior, she is doing it for the same reasons as the infant. There are many reflex-like or innate responses an infant shows that it loses as it matures (for example, the grasping and sucking reflexes). When an adult shows the same behavior (for example, grasping and sucking), it does not follow that the adult is showing an innate behavior. In fact, it is very unlikely that the adult is doing it for the same reasons. Further, since what adults judge to be physically attractive has a high degree of averageness, then the infant preference for such faces seems explicable as simply a preference for averageness or prototypes.[64] These are preferred because they help with information processing. With other stimuli, such as dot patterns and speech sounds, infants are able quickly to form an awareness of prototypes. Moreover, it seems that after exposure to a mere 16 to 32 faces, an infant can construct the idea of an average or a prototypical face. The infant preference for attractive faces (that is, for prototypical faces), can then be seen as merely an information-processing mechanism.[65]

But where, then, do older persons' ideas about physical attraction come from? Are they also merely a preference for prototypes? The situation here, I would argue, is more complex. This is because as we grow and begin to understand the human condition, physical appearance takes on different meanings for us. These meanings reflect our existential situation. We learn very early, for example, that sickness, old age, and death are waiting for each of us. This causes anxiety because it points to our own vulnerability and demise. The universality of this awareness is enshrined in the story of the life of the ancient Indian philosopher Gautama Buddha. In this story it is his contact with these existential truths that causes him to set off in search of an answer to our suffering. But it is because of this anxiety, I would argue, that features that are indicative of, or even a reminder of, lack of health, lack of youth, and oncoming death are ones that people prefer to avoid, even unconsciously. They are therefore seen to be physically unattractive. Features that are typically associated with physical unattractiveness, whether or not they actually indicate a lack of health, lack of youth, or oncoming death, have just these associations. Accordingly, they are also seen to be physically unattractive. On the other hand, those features that indicate health, youth, and liveliness direct our gaze away from sickness, old age, and death and so are seen to be physically attractive. They point to life and all its joys.

Although it might seem paradoxical, it is for similar reasons that an older individual who is well past his or her youth can also be seen as physically attractive. For the older man or woman who is seen to be physically attractive is just that person who, despite his or her age, is nevertheless seen to be healthy, in good shape, and lively. This also displays a fortitude that points to the joy of living. Since, as I argued earlier, there are indistinct areas where the difference between physical and sexual attraction might become unclear, this explanation might also account for some aspects of sexual attraction.

I have now laid out the various features of sexual attraction: its relation to other forms of interpersonal attraction, its tie to physical appearance, its distinction from sexual desire and physical attraction, and the nature of allure, which lies at its core. I have, however, said little about the human relationships in which sexual attraction takes place. But an understanding of how sexual attraction manifests itself in these relationships is vital for understanding sexual attraction itself. This is because, as I said at the beginning of the section on allure, allure singles out another person by directing our awareness to the other person's ability to attract us sexually. The sexually attractive person, however, is fundamentally entangled in the relationship we have to him or her. Therefore, the sexually attractive person is for me, and for the allure that I have for her, either a stranger, a friend, a romantic partner, or some such thing. To get a complete picture of the nature of allure, we must have an understanding of how allure operates in each of these relationships. It is to these relationships that I now turn.

TWO

Exchanging Glances

TYPES OF STRANGERS

One of the more peculiar aspects of sexual attraction is how easily it is elicited by strangers. This is peculiar because sexual attraction to another person is attraction to an intimate act of baring and caressing with that person. A stranger, however, is someone with whom one has no prior form of intimacy and whom one knows little or nothing about. This, it seems, is the essential feature of strangers, that is, their unknownness. Because of this, the idea of being sexually attracted to a stranger seems, on the face of it, odd. Why would one feel attracted to intimacy with an unknown person? If the sexual attraction did lead to its goal—namely, a sexual interaction—the person may react in any number of unexpected ways, ways that may be highly unpleasant or even dangerous. Further, because most of the strangers one sees, including those one finds alluring, have their clothes on, one remains fairly unsure as to how the fantasized bodily union would go. Maybe the feeling of his or her skin is not what one would imagine it to be. Maybe his or her genitals are not as attractive as one had expected them to be, or perhaps they do not feel as one imagined they would in the moment of an intimate caress. Or maybe, upon actually sinking one's teeth into the attractive person, one is filled with an unpleasant taste.

These sorts of problems are for the most part absent in sexual attraction to someone one knows or with whom one has had some form of physical closeness or intimacy. Here one has at least some idea of how the person would react in a sexual encounter. One might also be more aware of the physical features of the other person's body along with the experience of physical intimacy with that person's body. The sexual fantasies of allure will have more concrete images to build upon. Because of this, it would seem that sexual attraction would tend to keep at least to persons one knows. This, however, is far from the case. As is readily evident, sexual attraction to strangers runs rampant through people's lives.

Why, then, should this be the case? The answer can already be found in what was established in the last chapter, namely, that sexual attraction is fundamentally concerned with physical appearance. With this it is easily understandable that one can be sexually attracted to a stranger. For the physical appearance of a stranger is as evident as the physical appearance of people we know. Consequently, one can as easily be attracted to a stranger as to anyone else. Still, the dynamics of sexual attraction to a stranger are more complex than this. To get a picture of what is going on in this sort of sexual attraction, let us start by examining the idea of a stranger.

The first thing to notice here is that before sexual attraction to a stranger can take place, the stranger must normally be seen to be of the appropriate gender. For the heterosexual observer, the stranger is usually seen to be of the opposite sex, while for the homosexual observer the stranger should be of the same sex, and for the bisexual observer the stranger can be of either sex. Though, again, it is important to remember there can be degrees of homosexual or bisexual attraction. Therefore, the stranger who appears as sexually attractive must be someone who displays the gender to which one is sexually orientated. In addition to this distinction, there will be several degrees and types of strangers. Each one of these, I shall argue, presents himself or herself to our awareness in different ways and therefore affects the allure the stranger has for us.

What, then, are the different types of strangers? At the most basic level a stranger is someone whom one knows nothing about other than what one can observe. In the purest case a stranger will be someone whom one has seen but briefly for the first time. At this level there will be no interaction, not even eye contact, between oneself and the stranger. This probably constitutes the vast majority of strangers in many people's lives, at least in the lives of those who live or work in urban centers or other highly populated areas. This "unnoticing stranger," as I will call him or her, is someone who appears but briefly in one's field of observation, only suddenly then to disappear. Brevity is essential here because the longer one watches another person, the less of a stranger she seems to become. As the brevity begins to disappear, so does the initial experience of unknownness. As the seconds tick by, one begins to notice things one had not seen before. One might notice particular facial or bodily features, habitual movements, or gestures, all of which give one more material with which to form an impression of the person. Such an impression, however, need not be accurate. The important difference is merely that as one's observation of another person continues, one develops a sense of knowing more about the person. Yet for all this one has no way of knowing whether impressions formed through such exposure are accurate. When this is taken together with the fact that one has no interpersonal contact with the individual thus observed, then the person remains essentially a stranger, though of course the impressions one has formed may make the person seem less of a stranger.

A line is crossed, however, when interpersonal contact is made with the stranger. By "interpersonal contact" I am referring to the instant in which the unnoticing stranger suddenly notices the observer noticing him or her and, at the same time, the observer notices that his observation of the stranger is noticed by the stranger. In other words, both are simultaneously aware of each other's awareness of each other. At this point an unnoticing stranger becomes what I will call a "contacted stranger." The line that is crossed here is the line between the observation of an unknowing person and the mutual awareness that two strangers suddenly have of each other. Probably the most common behavior that results in the transition to this mutual awareness between strangers would be mutual gaze or eye contact. In eye contact the pupils of each person are aimed directly at the pupils of the other person. When this occurs, there is little doubt for each person that the other person has noticed him or her.

This suddenly brings in a new level to the observer's awareness of the stranger. Prior to this moment the stranger was unaware of being observed. As a result, his or her behavior took no or little account of the observer. With eye contact, however, this all suddenly changes and the observation by the observer becomes an interaction. This does not mean that the stranger's overt actions need change in any dramatic or even obvious way. It only means that the stranger's behavior is now carried out in the full awareness that he or she is being observed, along with the full awareness that the observer knows that the stranger knows he or she is being observed. The unknown state of the stranger loses its completeness, for the observer now knows that the stranger knows that the observer is watching him or her. Further, it is just this knowledge that, by creating an interpersonal relation, starts to remove the stranger's strangerness.

Although eye contact is one way of establishing such contact, it is not the only way. Another is what might be called peripheral-vision contact. In this case an observed person becomes aware through her peripheral vision that she is being observed. This is not mutual gaze or eye contact because there is no meeting of pupils. Nevertheless, peripheral vision can be sensitive enough to note one is being observed, though here it will depend more on reading behavioral cues. In such a case, an unnoticing stranger becomes aware he is being observed by noticing the observer "out of the corner of his eye," which does not mean looking directly at the observer's eyes but rather sensing the observer's activities on the periphery of his visual field. At the same time the person doing the observing becomes aware that the other person is aware of being observed and is observing him back through peripheral vision. In this moment each person is visually aware of each other's observation of him or her, though there is an asymmetry in their visual awareness of each other, with one having more direct visual contact than the other.

One could wonder how it is possible to know someone is using his or her peripheral vision to observe what one is doing. In the case of direct eye contact, there is no doubt that each knows mutual observation is taking place. But here, because the observed person is not looking directly back at the observer, it would seem that the observer cannot know if the observed person is aware of being observed. I think, however, we are normally sensitive enough to each other's behavior, especially eye behavior, to know when someone is using peripheral vision to observe us. When this happens the person's gaze seems to be nowhere in particular. It is much like when someone who is tired or daydreaming defocuses his or her eyes and gazes off into space. However, in this situation the eyes are more glassy and relaxed. In peripheral-vision use, the gaze, though to nowhere in particular, is more intense and fixed. One can see that the eyes are being held firmly in place in order to use the peripheral vision. There are also other telltale eye movements. For example, although the person in this case does not look directly at the other person, his or her eyes nevertheless may shift somewhat in direction of the person being observed. This shift, which can be back and forth—slightly toward the person being observed and then back to nowhere in particular—or held somewhat persistently toward the person being observed, betray the person's use of peripheral vision.

There are also other behaviors that seem to accompany peripheral-vision use. One obvious behavior is the stilling of bodily movements. This is done, I would suggest, in order to both hold the peripheral focus (if one can use such a term) on the person being observed and to attend to the indistinct and out-of-focus image that the observer is trying to concentrate on. In observing someone directly, the stilling of bodily movement is not necessary. One can easily observe another person directly when one is walking past or otherwise moving one's body. But in peripheral vision the image of the person one is trying to observe is indistinct and unclear. Therefore, bodily movement interferes with this use of peripheral vision. Because of this, someone using his or her peripheral vision to observe another will also tend to betray his observational activities by stilling his bodily movements.

The reason I use the word "betray" is because it seems obvious that, in these situations, the reason for the use of peripheral vision is that it enables a person to attempt to hide the fact that he is observing another person. But it is just this attempting to hide his awareness of the other person that distinguishes peripheral-vision contact from eye contact. For in attempting to hide his awareness, he makes it clear that he thinks the person he is observing is unaware of being observed. That is, he thinks his attempts to secretly observe the other person are successful. But in the situation I am describing, they are not successful. Consequently, peripheral-vision contact lacks the full reciprocal awareness that takes place in eye contact. In eye contact both parties know that each other knows that they are observing each other. In peripheral-vision contact the individual using peripheral vision is unaware that the person he is observing knows he is being observed. Because of this, it does not transform an unnoticing stranger to contacted stranger as fully as does direct eye contact.

Even so, it is worth pointing out that someone who, because of eye contact, is aware she is being observed can still attempt to hide this awareness from her observer. One way of doing this, it seems, is for her to immediately break eye contact with her observer by looking off to the side as if she were looking at other things. This common behavior, I would suggest, is an attempt by the person being observed to downplay the significance of the moment of eye contact by trying to get the observer to think that, although there was eye contact, it was hardly even noticed. By quickly moving her gaze on to other things, the observed person might hope the observer will think that the observer's eyes are merely just one (or two) of the many objects that the observed person is busy looking at, and therefore not so important after all.

The problem, however, is that the instant of eye contact is too salient to be sloughed off in this way. This is especially so when it occurs between strangers of the opposite sex or the gender appropriate for each other's sexual attraction and when at least one of them might see the other as sexually attractive. Eyes, especially sexually interested eyes, are never just two of the many objects one is busy looking at. It must be remembered, though, that despite all this interaction, which separates the contacted stranger from the unnoticing stranger, the contacted stranger remains a stranger. Very little is known about the contacted stranger.

Yet a further way that an unnoticing stranger can become a contacted stranger is through bodily contact. Although probably less common than eye or peripheral-vision contact, it nevertheless can be a way in which an unnoticing stranger is brought into contact with his or her observer. Such an event might well take place in a situation where strangers are crowded together, such as in an elevator, public transport, or at a gathering. Here one person might, because of the crowded situation, be brought into bodily contact with a stranger. Were one person aware of the other by, say, focusing on her feeling of his body pressed against hers, but that person not fully aware of her body pressed up against his (maybe he is distracted by other events or bodies), then the unaware person would essentially be an unnoticing stranger. That is, he would be an unaware stranger who was being observed (albeit with touch rather than vision) by an observer. Were such an unnoticing stranger then suddenly to become aware of the tactile observation—that is, that the touch of the other person's body was a form of observation—and further, were he to impart his awareness of the observation back to the observer (say, by moving in a way that communicated his awareness of being touched), then he would become a contacted stranger.

There is also, it should be noted, the stranger who lies somewhere between the noticing and contacted stranger. This is the stranger who, though having no interpersonal contact with a specific observer, is nevertheless acutely aware of being observed by people in general. This is the stranger who, for example, casually strolls past an observer without engaging in eye contact or even peripheral-vision contact. Even so, she makes it clear, through various self-conscious behaviors, that she wants people to notice her. The behaviors here might include stylized walking, gazing into nowhere while resolutely avoiding eye contact, talking on her mobile telephone a little too animatedly, or, if she is with her friends, laughing a little too loudly. This person is not a fully fledged unnoticing stranger because she is quite aware of being watched. On the other hand, she is not a fully contacted stranger because she has not established contact with the observer.

In addition to the unnoticing stranger and contacted stranger, there is also the stranger one has spotted on various earlier occasions, a person who could be termed the "seen-before stranger." This commonly happens when one notices the same unknown person waiting, for example, at the same bus stop each day, in the same shop at different times, or walking through the same neighborhood. What essentially distinguishes this type of stranger from the others is the sense of recognition one feels upon seeing him or her. This creates the peculiar experience of recognizing someone whom one does not know. This is peculiar because the sense of recognizing something normally carries with it the sense of familiarity. And the sense of familiarity, in turn, brings with it the idea that one has a knowledge of, experience with, and expectations about the thing with which one is familiar. But in the situation here, what one recognizes is a stranger, that is, someone with whom one has only a superficial familiarity and, consequently, no real experience or expectations. Rather, one simply recognizes the person's physical appearance.

Things, however, become more complex when we observe that the seen-before stranger comes in two forms, namely, the "seen-before unnoticing stranger" and the "seen-before contacted stranger." In the first case the stranger is someone whom one has seen on other occasions but with whom one has never had contact. In this case, the stranger might have passed by the observer at different times, perhaps in crowded circumstances, and yet never have noticed the observer noticing her. In the second case, the same sort of thing might have happened with the exception that the stranger at some point displays an awareness to the observer (most likely through eye contact) that she knows he is observing her. When the stranger displays this awareness after a point at which the observer has seen her more than once, she then transforms for the observer from a seen-before unnoticing stranger to a seen-before contacted stranger.

Consider, for example, the case of a man who described to me how each day he started his commuting at the same busy train station. One day he noticed a particular woman waiting at the same station. She, however, did not notice him watching her. Several days later he happened to spot her again waiting at the same station. This time, however, she seemed to notice him out of the corner of her eye and turned to look in his direction. Her eyes met his briefly, but she continued moving her eyes to look past him in an effort, he explained, to undo the contact that the brief eye contact had established. He saw her at the station a few times after that, sometimes with brief eye contact and other times with what he felt was an active avoidance of eye contact. In either case it was clear that her behavior had changed as she changed from a seen-before unnoticing stranger to a seen-before contacted stranger.

Yet a further type of stranger is the stranger with whom one has a brief interaction, that is, an interaction that is more than mere eye or body contact. The most common form of interaction here will probably be conversation, though conversation, at least in its face-to-face variety, will also include displays of body language and other forms of nonverbal communication. Other forms of purely nonverbal interaction are also possible. In addition, this "interacted-with stranger" can be someone whom one has not noticed before, or she can be someone who was previously an unnoticing stranger or a contacted stranger. In any case, the decisive feature is that one interacts and exchanges information with the person. The information exchanged need not take the form of self-disclosure, that is, verbal statements wherein both people purposively disclose biographical facts. It can merely be chit-chat about the weather, surroundings, or what have you. These sorts of interactions frequently serve purposes like gathering information about the stranger and attempting to manage the impression of oneself given to the stranger. This type of information gathering and presentation is achieved to a large degree through nonverbal communication. In such a case, things like proximity, orientation toward, or away from the other person, and opening or closing off one's body (as in opening or crossing one's arms or legs) are used to gather and send interpersonal messages about things like dominance, submission, friendliness, or hostility.[1]

For my purposes the important thing about this kind of exchange is that it has an effect on the stranger's strangerness as it presents itself to our awareness. That is, a stranger whom one is interacting and conversing with is in the process of quickly losing the feature of being a stranger. That is, as the interaction proceeds, the interacted-with stranger becomes better and better known. This can occur both through one's observation of the stranger's body language and through what the stranger communicates verbally. As the interaction progresses, one will learn more and more about the stranger's personality, dispositions, values, and so forth, or at least what the stranger wants one to think are his or her personality, dispositions, and values. The sociologist Erving Goffman, for example, gives an elaborate account of how people present each other with idealized versions of "fronts" in which they try to control how the other person sees them.[2] Despite this, having access to all of this quickly chips away at what one experiences as the strangerness of the stranger, eventually transforming him into an acquaintance.

It is nearly impossible to say, however, when exactly this transformation occurs. So many things will play in here that it will prove immensely difficult to find a clear line between the interacted-with stranger and the acquaintance. Things like the topic discussed, the presence of humor, the extent of eye contact, the degree of reciprocity, proximity, whether touching occurs and, if so, how it is received—all will work to affect one's sense of whether and to what degree the person remains a stranger, albeit an interacted-with stranger. Without being too precise, however, it would seem that after somewhere between 5 and 10 minutes of one-to-one effective interaction, one would no longer see the other person as a complete stranger. This would seem to be even more the case if, after having had such an interaction with the person, one meets the person a second or third time. In other words, there would be no such thing as a seen-before, interacted-with stranger. For being both "seen before" and "interacted with" would render the person no longer a stranger. Such a person would then be experienced as a casual acquaintance.

There are, of course, cases that challenge this, cases where one might intensively interact with the same stranger on different occasion but share little or no verbal communication. What I have in mind, which is in line with the focus of this book, is a case where two strangers meet regularly to have sex but say little to each other. A situation like this is portrayed in the film *Intimacy*, where the main character meets once a week to have sex with a woman he knows nothing about, not even her name. The two say next to nothing to each other, and after they have had sex, the woman promptly leaves.

The question that could be raised here is this: After the man has had sex with the woman, say even just once, does she remain a stranger to him? The fact that they have verbally shared no personal information with each other might tempt someone to conclude that they remain essentially strangers. However, verbal exchanges are only one way of acquiring personal information about another person. Because of the intensity and physical intimacy of sexual interaction, there is much that one can learn about another person in a sexual encounter, especially if one is sensitive to the other individual's body language and other nonverbal communications. The way the person responds to the increasing sexual arousal, his or her active or passive disposition, displays of dominance, submission, hostility, or kindness, all come together in the act of having sex to paint a distinct picture of aspects of the individual's personality. Because of this, it seems wrong to me to say the woman remains a stranger after the man has had sex with her. This seems especially so after they have had sex two or more times. In this situation, the woman has then moved on to being a sort of acquaintance. So here, too, there appears to be no such thing as a seen-before, interacted-with stranger.

This is not meant to be an exhaustive account of the forms that strangers can take in our awareness, and there will no doubt be subtle variations, degrees, and combinations of the types of strangers I have described. I do feel, however, that the account presented here captures the principal ways in which we experience strangers. Let us now see how sexual attraction to strangers takes place.

THE ALLURE OF STRANGERS

Sexual attraction to strangers is common and powerful. But why should this be the case, especially when strangers are people we know next to nothing about? One reason is that, as I mentioned earlier, sexual attraction is concerned with physical appearance. But this is also true for sexual attraction to nonstrangers, for example, to friends and romantic partners. Yet it is also evident that sexual attraction operates differently when it emanates from strangers rather than nonstrangers. This is because sexual attraction is not unaffected by the person it comes from. It does, after all, have its origin in the sexually attractive person. Consequently, the way we experience the person who gives off the attraction will influence how the attraction appears in our awareness. To see how this works, there is no other way than to turn to an examination of the allure that strangers emanate toward those who are sexually attracted to them.

As was established in the last chapter, allure consists of the sense of being drawn toward a sexually attractive other, a sense of helplessness in thus being drawn, and a sexual fantasy concerning a physical intimacy with the person one is being drawn toward. In the case where the person one is attracted to is a stranger, each of these elements will be experienced in a distinct way. These elements will further be affected according to the type of stranger one is attracted to. How, then, is the allure of the stranger experienced?

One of the central elements of the experience of a stranger is the unknownness we feel upon observing him or her, for strangers suddenly appear to us out of nowhere. One is aware, at some level, that the stranger has a background, a family, plans, concerns, and so forth. But none of this is known to us in the moment we observe the stranger. Nor can we search our memory to bring the information forth, as we can when we meet, say, an old acquaintance. All we are presented with is the physical appearance of the stranger. Again, we can speculate and try, Sherlock Holmes–like, to garner clues from what we immediately see. Perhaps the person's behavior or clothing suggests something about him or her, but such suggestions remain essentially unconfirmed conjecture. What the stranger is for the observer is simply as he appears in the moment. Beyond that, there is nothing to the stranger for the observer. It is almost like the stranger suddenly materializes in the moment he or she is perceived, only to dematerialize when he or she is gone from view. This leads in most cases to varying degrees of indifference, though, of course, different aspects of strangers may catch our attention. All of this changes, however, when the stranger is seen to be sexually attractive.

With the unnoticing stranger, the allure entices one forward in a purely impersonal way. Lacking any interpersonal contact with the stranger, one experiences the physical appearance of the stranger as all that is definite about him or her. When the stranger who is observed is seen to be sexually attractive, this has a powerful effect on the observer. This is because the observer's awareness of the sexual attraction is undiluted with other features of the stranger. Because there is no contact between the observer and the stranger, the sexual attraction that emanates from the stranger reaches out to the observer, as it were, all by itself. If there were interpersonal contact, then ideas about what the stranger is thinking or what view the stranger has of the observer would also find their way into the observer's awareness. Although such thoughts would have little to do with the sexual attraction itself, depending on the content of these thoughts they may well direct awareness away from the sexual attraction, taking the observer's thought off in other directions.

With the unnoticing stranger there is less chance of that. Here both the sense of being drawn toward the person and the sense of helplessness at being drawn have a pureness about them that, depending on the degree of sexual attractiveness, can give the allure of the stranger a stark quality. This quality can be further heightened by the nature of the sexual fantasies that help make up the allure. For the observer of the unnoticing stranger, these fantasies will occur in the state of noncontact with the stranger. Consequently, they will tend to have more free play.

Looking at sexual fantasies that take place outside of the experience of allure, it is evident that they can occur in at least two distinct ways. As noted, they can take place when one is alone, forming images that are independent of other people's immediate actions, or they can occur during sexual or other types of encounters. Here the images are typically tied loosely to the actual encounter. For example, a woman who is having sexual intercourse with her partner might fantasize that she is a prostitute or that her partner is another man she knows from work. Therefore, although she is fantasizing about these aspects of the encounter, her fantasy is still tied to the fact that she is having sexual intercourse.

Interestingly enough, a similar distinction can be found with the fantasies that appear within the allure of strangers. This is the distinction between fantasies about the unnoticing stranger and fantasies about the contacted stranger. For there is a sense in which one is alone when observing the unnoticing stranger (only the observer is observing), whereas one is not alone when observing a contacted stranger (both are observing each other). In the former case the fantasy takes place outside an interaction, in the latter case the fantasy occurs in the midst of contact with the stranger, or at least shortly thereafter. This makes the fantasy about the unnoticing stranger a bit like a solitary sexual fantasy, and the fantasy about the contacted stranger somewhat like the fantasy during a sexual encounter, but only so far as it is a fantasy that takes place in the midst of an interaction. Here there is no sexual encounter. And just as a sexual fantasy engaged in alone would seem typically less constrained by the circumstances, so is a sexual fantasy in the allure of the unnoticing stranger less constrained by the circumstances. In neither case is the observer simultaneously interacting with another person. This means the observer is free from the possible distractions or influences that such an interaction must involve. In certain situations this might give the fantasy more scope.

To see how a fantasy in the allure to an unnoticing stranger can appear, consider the verses from a poem "Leg in the Subway" by Oscar Williams:

When I saw the woman's leg on the floor of the subway train,
Protrude beyond the panel (while her body overflowed my
  mind's eye),
When I saw the pink stocking, black shoe, curve bulging with
  warmth,
The delicate etching of the hair behind the flesh-colored gauze,
When I saw the ankle of Mrs. Nobody going nowhere for a nickel,
When I saw this foot motionless on the moving motionless floor,
My mind caught on a nail of a distant star, I was wrenched out
Of the reality of the subway ride, I hung in a socket of distance:
And this is what I saw:
The long tongue of the earth's speed was licking the leg,
Upward and under and around went the tongue of speed:
It was made of flesh invisible, it dripped the saliva of miles:
It drank moment, lit shivers of insecurity in niches between bones. . . .[3]

In this description we are first given a detailed account of the unnoticing stranger, or rather part of the stranger, that captures the observer's sexual interest: a stockinged leg that reaches out from behind a panel. Stockinged female legs whose owners are hidden are a well-known inducer of male of sexual attraction and, as a result, are commonly portrayed. In the film *Derailed*, for example, it is shapely nylon-encased legs, also in black shoes (high heels), also sticking out from behind a panel, and also on the floor of a train, that capture the main character's attention (along with the attention of all the other male passengers). This sets his attraction in motion and induces him to approach the stranger. In the poem, the leg owner's status as an unnoticing stranger is expressed by being called "Mrs. Nobody going nowhere." The observer's sudden experience of the power of the attraction and his helplessly being drawn are captured in the lines "My mind caught on a nail of a distant star, I was wrenched out/Of the reality of the subway ride, I hung in a socket of distance."

In a way the stranger with the lovely leg is the star whose nail he is caught on: she is the twinkling star whose sheer prominence pulls him helplessly into her gravitational field. His mind is, after all, caught on the star's nail. This is why he is "wrenched out of the reality of the subway ride." For in the reality of the subway ride, she is over there and he is over here and, further, he is not moving toward her. Nevertheless, the allure of the stranger's leg wrenches him out of this reality by seeming to wrench him toward her. This might well be what he means by saying, "I was hung in a socket of distance": he was helplessly caught by her sexual attractiveness (hanging on the nail of her star), feeling himself pulled toward her but nevertheless being aware that he was at a distance from her, as if suspended in a bubble or socket.

The fantasized intimate joining with the unnoticing stranger, or rather her curvaceous and warm leg (though her imagined body does overflow into his mind's eye), comes in the form of a fantasy of licking the leg "upward and under and around." He does not say that it is him licking the leg, but rather the "long tongue of earth's speed" or the "tongue of speed." Although the meaning of this poetical expression is unclear, I think it can be easily understood within this picture of allure. Since the woman is much like a star who has caught him in its gravitational field, pulling him toward her, he can be seen as much like earth that is caught in the gravitational pull of the sun (which is a star). And just like the earth, though being pulled toward the sun never falls into it, so he, who is pulled toward the stockinged leg, is nevertheless "hung in a socket." Still, he fantasizes himself reaching out quickly across the distance—with the long tongue of earth's speed—to lick the stranger's leg all over. That it is both his tongue and yet a fantasized tongue is shown by the fact that "It was made of flesh invisible." "It dripped the saliva of miles" is just his drooling over the delicious leg that is both so close and yet so far. Further, in his sexual fantasy, the leg responds to his licking by having "shivers of insecurity in niches between bones."

Although this sort of imagery might seem odd, sexual symbolism seems to be a not uncommon feature of sexual fantasies, both in the fantasies of allure and in other sexual fantasies. For example, while having sexual intercourse with her partner, one woman had the fantasy that she was a massive tree—"the tree of life" as she called it—with roots traveling down to the core of the earth and branches and leaves reaching up to the sun. She fantasized that her partner was the sun and that as they had sex she could feel his life energy coursing through her.[4]

Turning now to the contacted stranger, it is evident that allure takes on a somewhat different appearance. This is because a stranger becomes a contacted stranger only when both the stranger and the observer are aware that they are observing each other. As I mentioned, the most common form of this exchange of awareness is eye contact. As with any two people, whether they are strangers or not, eye contact can signal many things. Depending on how it is done, eye contact, and especially ways of intensifying or breaking eye contact, can send various signals: glaring intensely at someone can signal aggression, glistening eyes can signal adoration or intense liking, breaking eye contact downward can display submissiveness, while breaking eye contact sideways or avoiding eye contact can show dominance or indifference.[5]

However, with the transformation of an alluring and unnoticing stranger into an alluring and contacted stranger, the decisive feature is simply eye contact in any form. Here it is evident that the eye contact can affect the allure in at least two ways. First, by looking at the stranger directly in the eyes, the observer is given a further angle on the stranger's physical appearance, namely, the appearance of the stranger's eyes. For although one can see another person's eyes even if there is no eye contact with the person, nothing compares to the view of someone's eyes when they are viewed in full eye contact. Eyes are a basic feature of someone's sexual attractiveness. Although true for both men and women, this seems especially true for women, whose eyes are normally larger than men's. Further, the whites of a woman's eyes are also more prominent than a man's, providing more of a frame for the display of the irises.

The widespread use of eye makeup by women, which goes all the way back to ancient Egypt, seems to reflect an awareness of this natural feature of women's eyes by trying to exaggerate it. Eye makeup, especially eyeliner and mascara, does this by framing the whites of the eyes, which in turn frame the irises, and thus underscoring the largeness of the female eyes while accentuating their more prominent white sections. Eye shadow provides the same effect by providing an even larger frame in which to set off the whites of the eyes. But it can also serve the further function of drawing attention to the irises by mimicking their color. Even when eye shadow is a different color from the irises, it still seems to draw attention to them. This is because the irises are the colored part of the eye (be they blue, gray, green, hazel, or brown) lying between the colorless white of the eye and colorless black of the pupil. Because of this, colored eye lids easily accentuate or remind us of colored irises. Colored eyelids also have the purpose of keeping the observer continuously aware of—and attracted to—this colorful aspect of the eyes. When the eyes are open, it is the irises that perform this feat; when they are closed, the colored eyelids take over. Consequently, even though any interaction involving eye contact will include numerous instants of blinking, the hiding of the colored irises is in the same instant replaced by a display of the colored eyelids. It is almost as if the blinking eyes are saying, "I know the colored irises are momentarily gone, but please enjoy these colored eyelids until they return." It is also noteworthy that a common female behavior in courtship, or even in simple cross-sex interactions, is breaking eye contact by gazing downward. This is typically seen to be a submissive gesture, much like bowing the head. It is one that colored eyelids not only bring attention to but also seem to celebrate with their colorfulness.

In addition to the attractive appearance of the whites of the eyes and the irises during eye contact, there is also the attractive appearance of the pupils. A major feature here is their size. Research has shown that during eye contact, large pupils are seen to be more sexually attractive than small pupils. In a much cited study, male subjects were shown pairs of pictures of the same female and asked to rate which was most attractive. The pictures were identical except for the fact that in one picture the pupils of the woman had been altered to look larger. Although the men in the study could not say what the difference was between the two pictures (they had not consciously noticed the different size of pupils), they nevertheless rated the picture with the large pupils to be more attractive.[6] The results of this study have been replicated several times.[7]

Some people have tried to explain this by suggesting that since large pupils show an interest in what is being viewed, during eye contact they show an interest in the person being viewed. As a result, we will tend to find large pupils attractive because they show an interest in us. This explanation, however, at least as far as sexual attraction goes, strikes me as implausible. One reason for this is that when similar studies are done on women's responses to pupil size in men, the results have been inconsistent.[8] If the explanation is strictly that large pupils show interest, then it seems women should also rate men with large pupils as more attractive. Further, as I argued earlier, sexual attraction is basically connected to physical appearance, not to personality or dispositions, which include the disposition to be interested in the attracted person. A woman is not sexually attracted to a man's masculine physique, small buttocks, and scent because it shows that he is interested in her. Nor is a man sexually attracted to an hourglass figure and female way of walking because it shows she is attracted to him.

Of course, the fact that someone you are sexually attracted to is likewise sexually attracted to you carries other implications with it. It implies, for example, that you stand a better chance of achieving the goal of your sexual attraction, namely, to have sex with the person. It also implies the slight chance of achieving a long-term relationship with the person, if that is what you also want. But such considerations are not the stuff of sexual attraction.

A better explanation might be that large pupils simply look better. They might do so by making the eyes look more balanced and supplying a clearer contrast with the whites of the eyes. Or it might be that large pupils make the eyes look bigger. This would explain why men are more consistent in rating larger pupils more attractive. For having larger pupils would increase a woman's sexual attractiveness by exaggerating the already feminine feature of large eyes. In the case of men's appearance, it might increase their sexual attractiveness, though not as clearly as women's pupils do, by making them appear less excessively masculine. This fits with the evidence that women tend to prefer more feminine-looking male faces over stereotypically rugged-looking male faces.[9] This is a finding that has been shown to exist in such distinct cultures as Scottish, Japanese, and tribes of the Amazon.[10] Female preference for less excessively masculine features appears in other areas, too. Therefore, although chest and body hair is clearly a masculine trait, women across different cultures express a preference for males with less body hair.[11]

The second way in which eye contact can affect the allure of a stranger is not by giving a better angle on the physical appearance of the stranger, but rather by working directly on the components of the stranger's allure. Thus, when I am under the sway of an unnoticing stranger's allure, I feel myself being drawn helplessly toward an intimate physical contact with her. When, however, the situation suddenly alters and eye contact is made, I am immediately swept into a union of mutual awareness with the now contacted stranger. In the case of the sexually attractive stranger, this creates the sense of being drawn forward into the stranger's awareness. I enter the stranger's awareness in the sense that I suddenly "peer into" the stranger, as it were, discerning myself as the content of her awareness. This creates the sense of being drawn toward her, thus accentuating the experience of feeling pulled toward her, an experience that was already there before the moment of eye contact. It was present in the allure that I felt for her even as an unnoticing stranger.

Furthermore, eye contact intensifies the helplessness experienced in allure. This is because as soon as the stranger looks into my eyes, she will see my interest in her, an interest that she will most likely understand to be sexual attraction. This immediately intensifies my sense of being drawn toward her because now it is not only I who am aware of my sexual attraction toward her, but she is also aware. Moreover, and this is the important point, I am aware that she is aware of my sexual attraction toward her. Thus,

I am made doubly aware of the helpless state I am in: I am aware of it from my point of view and also aware that she knows this about me. In addition, the fact that she is aware of my sexual attraction seems to take my sexual attraction to her even further out of my control.

The experience of helplessness during eye contact is also something that is discussed by the existentialist philosopher Jean-Paul Sartre.[12] For Sartre, "the look" (as he calls the moment of eye contact) is an instance in which two people experience each other's freedom. What I experience in the look, according to Sartre, is the other person's freedom to construe me how he or she will, just as the other person experiences my freedom similarly to construe him or her. The freedom here comes from the fact that I have no control over what the other person is thinking about me, nor does he have any control over what am thinking about him. This leads to a conflict, or perhaps a staring contest, in which each person is trying to get the other to experience himself or herself as an object before his or her gaze. In trying to get the other person to do this, I am trying to cancel out my contestant's freedom by making him or her into a mere object. This is an attempt to escape the sense of helplessness that each person feels in the gaze of the other.

Although this exchange clearly happens in moments of eye contact, it is a different phenomenon from the one I am discussing. For Sartre, the look is confined to neither strangers nor sexual awareness. The account of eye contact that I am presenting is an account of an exchange between an observer and an alluring stranger. It is therefore one that takes place within sexual awareness. The helplessness that is experienced by the observer in this moment does not concern the stranger's freedom. It is rather concerns the sense of being magnetically pulled toward the stranger while at the same time having this sense intensified by the observer's awareness that the stranger is aware of his sexual attraction toward her.

I just said that when the alluring stranger establishes eye contact with her observer, she will most likely interpret his gaze as one of sexual attraction. The question of how someone might know that a brief moment of eye contact signals sexual attraction is an interesting one. Although there has been much research on eye contact and eye movements in the laboratory, little work has been done in the field on sexual attraction and eye contact between opposite-sex strangers. My suspicion, however, is that in most situations, when someone notices an opposite-sex stranger observing him or her, the default interpretation given to the stranger's gaze is one of sexual attraction. In other words, in the absence of any evidence to the contrary, an opposite-sex person's gaze will be taken by the other person to mean that the observer is showing sexual attraction. (And it is important to remember here that sexual attraction can be of different degrees, anything from very mild to intense.) Other behaviors of the observer, such as persistent or repeated eye contact, smiling, or bodily displays, could then be seen to support the sexual intent of the eye contact.

Finally, eye contact can affect the allure of a stranger by providing the observer with a sort of foreshadowing of the fantasized physical contact. Although eye contact is not physical contact, it is nevertheless a type of contact with the person observed. Therefore, when I am under the sway of an unnoticing stranger's allure, I feel myself being drawn helplessly toward an intimate physical contact with her. When, however, the situation suddenly alters and eye contact is made, I am immediately swept into a union of mutual awareness with the stranger. This gives me a sense of contact with the stranger, which can easily become symbolic of the fantasized joining of my body with hers. In this way eye contact with a sexually attractive stranger can stoke the fires of the stranger's allure. It does this by providing the sexual fantasy of allure with more material, albeit symbolic material.

That the moment of eye contact in sexual attraction to a stranger is a significant one is perhaps shown by the popularity of the song "Strangers in the Night," made famous by Frank Sinatra. For it is in this song that this moment and its relation to allure is celebrated. Of further interest is that the song not only refers to eye contact in the allure of a stranger, but it also more or less follows the progression from an unnoticed stranger, to a contacted stranger, to an interacted-with stranger, ending where the person is no longer a stranger. The song starts with the well-known lines:

> Strangers in the night exchanging glances
> Wond'ring in the night what were the chances
> We'd be sharing love before the night was through.

There is, to be sure, a metaphorical sense in which all strangers are more or less strangers in the night. For the night is shrouded in darkness, and darkness symbolizes the unknown. Consequently, the phrase "strangers in the night," though perhaps referring to the point of time where particular strangers find themselves, could also be a way of emphasizing the unknownness of strangers.

In "exchanging glances" the strangers make eye contact and become for each other contacted strangers. If we now consider this moment from the point of view of one of the strangers—the one who is allured (and perhaps they both are allured by each other)—then the "wond'ring in the night" seems to refer to the moment, in exchanging glances, in which the observer is aware that the stranger is aware of the observer's sexual attraction toward her. This intensifies the sense of being drawn to the stranger, leading to a wondering about what the end result of such a sensation might be. What the sensation of being pulled is hinting at, of course, is the physical intimacy of the observer and the stranger. This is conjured up in the sexual fantasy of allure, here the fantasized "sharing love before the night was through." Although "sharing love" might seem to refer to the feelings of love, the fact that the love might be shared "before the night was through" suggests that a less ambiguous expression might be "*making* love before the night was through."

The next verse, which is addressed directly to the stranger, says,

Something in your eyes was so inviting
Something in your smile was so exciting
Something in my heart told me I must have you.

These lines repeat similar ideas to those given in the first verse. Thus, in the exchanging of glances, the observer also sees something so inviting in the stranger's eyes. This "so inviting" refers, I would argue, to the intensification of the stranger's allure that is achieved through eye contact. "Inviting" is a good word because it places the allure in the stranger herself. Her allure invites or pulls the observer toward her. The next line, "something in you smile was so exciting," would seem also to refer to the same intensification achieved through eye contact (for eyes are also part of a smile). Though "exciting" does not directly refer to the sensation of being helplessly pulled toward the attractive stranger, it could easily refer to the sexual excitement that might accompany such a sensation.

The final line can be understood in several ways. However, it is natural enough to see it as referring to the fantasized joining that is the third element in allure. This is because the "something in my heart told me" can, in this context, refer to how the observer understands the experience of allure. Even though the allure of someone is sensed as coming from that person, an observer can nevertheless reflect over the sensation. Also, the phrase "I must have you" can be naturally interpreted to mean "I must have sex with you," or "I must have any physically intimate joining with you."

Shortly after this are the lines "we were strangers in the night up to the moment when we said our first hello." This is the point at which the contacted stranger transforms into an interacted-with stranger. (In the song there is no account of the seen-before stranger, for as the song tells us,

"Ever since that night we've been together.") Although I have argued that an interacted-with stranger is still a stranger (and thus, in a sense, a stranger in the night), it depends on what the import is of "said our first hello." If this refers to an instance of chatting and interaction that goes on for more than 5 or 10 minutes, then although at the beginning of their conversation they were interacted-with strangers, after they said their first hello they were no longer strangers (in the night).

Before we leave the allure of the contacted stranger, it is worthwhile to say something about the alluring stranger who is contacted, not with eye contact but with physical contact. As with any strangers, this form of contact between an observer and an alluring stranger would seem to be less common, probably occurring mainly in crowded environments. When this happens we could imagine it occurring in a similar way to when eye contact takes place between an observer and an unnoticing stranger. Imagine, for example, that a woman who is in a crowded room finds herself pressed up against various people. At one point she becomes aware that, because of the crowded conditions, a man's leg is inadvertently pressing into hers. Further, imagine that she then begins to notice the sexual attractiveness of the firm and muscular thigh gently pushing into her.

Although this idea of sexual attractiveness experienced through touch might seem initially odd, it should be obvious that not uncommonly we experience sexual attraction in just this way: the smoothness of someone's skin, the silkiness of his or her hair, the heaviness of her breasts, can all work to give rise to the person's allure. The unusual aspect of the case I am considering is that it takes place with a stranger. For strangers are not usually in the sort of physical contact that enables one or the other to experience sexual attraction through touch. Nevertheless, as shown in this example, it is easily imaginable.

Now, if the man is not aware that the woman is aware of his thigh, then, at this point—the point where she starts to feel sexual attraction to him—the man becomes for her an alluring unnoticing stranger. But now let us imagine that the man becomes not only aware of the woman's thigh, but also that the woman is aware of his thigh and, further, that she is aware that he is aware of her thigh against his. Perhaps some subtle movement of her thigh, maybe a tensing or slight pulling away of her body, indicates this to him. In this instant the man becomes an alluring contacted stranger for the woman.

In addition to progressing from an unnoticing stranger to a contacted stranger, an unnoticing stranger can also become, as stated earlier, a seen-before stranger, either a seen-before contacted stranger or a seen-before unnoticing stranger. In the case of an alluring stranger, this has the effect of presenting the observer with what might be called a repetitive attractiveness of the same person. In the case of an alluring stranger I have only seen for the first time, the allure is more or less constant, continually flowing out from the stranger as she remains in my gaze. There are, of course, exceptions to this, as in the situation in which one is seated near such a stranger on an extended airplane flight or train ride. Here the allure might begin to abate as the minutes or hours go by, but then it might take up again as one looks up from one's book to notice her again. In this sense, however, the stranger seen for the first time might slowly become something of a seen-before stranger.

In any case, the seen-before stranger has the effect of reinstituting a previous allure. This can create, I would argue, the powerful sensation of feeling oneself once again under a recognized allure. Because allure has a sense of helplessness to it, this will naturally create the sensation of once again being helpless before the same person's allure. And just as a series of waves that repeated beat against a wall will eventually cause the wall to give way, so will repeated waves of allure lead to the sensation of feeling that one is about to give way. Give way to what? To the pull of the seen-before stranger's allure. This would suggest that the allure of the seen-before stranger is, generally, an increased allure, though this will naturally depend on various factors. Things like the stranger's subsequent appearance, the conditions under which the stranger is seen, and the condition of the observer might all work to influence the seen-before stranger's allure.

The idea that a seen-before stranger will, even under the best conditions, tend to gain an increase in his or her allure seems challenged, however, by what is known as the Coolidge effect. The Coolidge effect refers to the tendency in many species for a male to be sexually stimulated by the presence of new female partner. The appearance of a new female leads to a renewal of sexual activity in an otherwise sexually satiated male. A male rat, for example, will mate with a female rat a few times before becoming satiated and wandering away. However, if a new female is presented to him, he is suddenly satiated no longer, seems strongly attracted to the new female, and begins a new round of mating.[13]

Many researchers have interpreted this effect as an evolutionary adaptation that enables a male to have a higher chance of impregnating more females and thus leaving more offspring. Others, however, point out that after the first ejaculation, the animal's sperm count is drastically reduced. This, along with the fact that even though the male continues to mate with new females, frequently no sperm is left in the female's reproductive tract, suggests that the Coolidge effect might well not result in more impregnations.[14] Further, although this phenomenon seems to be most common among male animals, it has also been shown to exist in the females of some species. Clearly, however, a female engaging in repetitive matings with new males does not increase her chances of more impregnations. She might increase her own chances of a single impregnation, but then why do not the females of other species also show this behavior? There may well be other evolutionary reasons for the females of these specifies showing the Coolidge effect, but in either case it might simply be a specific expression of a more generalized interest in novelty.[15] It seems worth noting here that one of the species in which the female shows the Coolidge effect is the golden hamster, an animal well known for its curiosity and high interest in novelty.

The Coolidge effect becomes even more interesting when it is noted that something like it appears to occur in human sexual interaction. Therefore, although there seem to be no studies on this, it does appear that a man who has just finished having sex with a woman (has ejaculated, lost his erection, and feels satiated) would be more likely to resume his sexual activities if a new women were suddenly to appear and make herself sexually available to him.

This tendency in the Coolidge effect—namely, to be stimulated by the presence of a new and possible sexual partner—does not just refer to the stimulation that takes place in sexual interaction, but also to that of the sexual attraction that can lead up to sexual interaction. For my purposes, then, the relevant question is whether the Coolidge effect has any effect on allure. And here we see the relevance of the question of the allure of the seen-before stranger. This is because the seen-before stranger is not a novel stimulus. If the Coolidge effect has an effect on the allure of strangers, then it would seem that the seen-before stranger would be experienced as having less allure than he or she had when he or she was a stranger seen for the first time. Therefore, in the example mentioned earlier of the man who saw a woman stranger on various occasions at a train station, if the Coolidge effect was working here, then it would appear that in the subsequent times he saw her she should start to lose her allure for him.

In discussing this issue there is an interesting study that should be considered. In this study, men were shown a series of pictures of female strangers and asked to rate them in terms of sexual attractiveness. The pictures that a subject rated as highly attractive were then mixed into another group of pictures that were then also shown to the man. This time subjects were asked once again to rate the pictures for their attractiveness. The results showed that the pictures that were rated as highly attractive in the first showing were not rated as highly when they were viewed the second time. When, however, the same procedure was done with women viewing pictures of men, the results were the opposite. That is, the pictures the women had viewed before were, on the second viewing, rated at a higher level of attractiveness than they were rated on the first viewing.[16]

If we think of these results in terms of the Coolidge effect, it looks like men are showing the Coolidge effect while women are not. Men show the Coolidge effect here, it could be argued, because in rating pictures of women as less attractive on the second viewing, they are responding to the fact that the woman in the photograph is no longer a novel stimulus. In the same way, it could be argued that the female subjects in the study are not showing the Coolidge effect and, indeed, are showing something opposite. For rather than losing attraction to a no longer novel stimulus (a man's picture they had seen before), they in fact become more attracted to it. This in turn might be interpreted to mean that, for men, a stranger seen for the first time loses something of her allure when she becomes a seen-before stranger, while for women such a transition increases the stranger's allure.

There are, however, various considerations that count against this interpretation. What makes me most wary of this view is that men, in real life, do not seem at all to lose interest in an alluring stranger simply because they have seen her before. She was gorgeous the first time she was spotted, and, if she really is gorgeous, the second time she is spotted one can only sigh and think, as the song puts it, "There she goes again!" Further, seeing her on subsequent occasions will probably enable the man to note more of her attractive features. Or, if she is wearing different clothes, these might serve to accentuate different sexually attractive aspects of her physical appearance.

If this is true, then it shows what is wrong with using the mentioned study as an indication of a male Coolidge effect with seen-before strangers. Photographs of faces are two-dimensional motionless representations of only one part of the body. They do not break into a smile, flash their eyes, or toss their hair. They have no height, figure, or way of walking. It is then understandable that a man seeing such a picture for the second time might become less interested in it and so rate it as less attractive than he did the first time.

But what, then, about the results for the women? If what I have just said is correct, why, then, did the women rate the same picture as more attractive the second time? One explanation could simply be that, as I have been arguing, the seen-before stranger tends to give off an increased allure. But because of the nature of the seen-before stranger—cropped photographs—this seems implausible for the reasons just given. A more likely explanation follows from something I argued in the last chapter, namely, that women are often socialized to consider sexual partners in terms of long-term relationships. Therefore, it might well be that although the female subjects were asked to rate the pictures of the men according to their sexual attractiveness, the idea of attractiveness as a long-term partner sneaked its way into their evaluations. One of the things that is important in such relationships is that one has a sense of familiarity with one's partner. Consequently, upon seeing the picture a second time, there was a sense of familiarity that was not there the first time. As a result, the picture was rated as more attractive (as long-term partner) when it was viewed the second time.

This brings us to the allure of the interacted-with stranger. From the point of view of sexual attraction, this sort of brief encounter serves at least two purposes. First, it gives access to more information about the stranger's sexual attractiveness. While interacting with the stranger, one is able to observe more closely the features of the person whom one finds sexually attractive, while at the same time to discover new features that were not evident before the interaction. Therefore, because such an interaction allows one to be in close proximity to the stranger, one is able to examine various facial and bodily features more closely. One also will have access to other features that might not have been available earlier, say, the scent of the person, the color or clarity of his or her eyes, and the sound of his or her voice. All this has little to do with any verbal statements or disclosures the person might make during the conversation. In this regard, the role of the conversation serves to provide one with an opportunity to assess further the stranger's sexual attractiveness. If this closer observation leads to an evaluation of the stranger as even more sexually attractive, then it will be felt as an intensification of the stranger's allure.

The second purpose will be that of allowing the allure of the stranger to work its magic. For in continuing to interact with the stranger, one allows oneself to become immersed in the stranger's allure. This is because the allure of the stranger does not disappear simply because one starts interacting with him or her. Rather, it continues to pull one helplessly toward its goal of an intimate bodily joining. Although it is unclear, my discussions with my students and others on this point suggest that the allure operates in a way similar to how it does with the seen-before stranger. In that case the repeated sightings of a sexually attractive stranger have the effect of making one feel one is about to give way to the pull of the allure. In the case of the interacted-with stranger, the allure of the stranger does not occur in repetitive waves but rather works on the observer as a constant force, much like the continuous pressure of a body of water on a dike or the wall of a dam.

However, numerous other things are usually happening in such an interaction. These can complicate the interaction. This is because in the case of sexual attraction to an interacted-with stranger, there is frequently more at stake than assessing the stranger's sexual attractiveness. The reason is that with the advent of interaction, all sorts of other possibilities suggest themselves. One such possibility is that of the fantasized sexual intimacy with the stranger being realized. That is, in the allure that the observer feels for the stranger, there will appear the element of an imagined sexual interaction with the stranger. With the beginning of the interaction, that fantasized physical intimacy, or at least a version of it, seems to become more possible.

Of course, a sexual interaction between the observer and the alluring stranger was always possible. But before this possibility had a realistic chance of becoming actual, some sort of interaction would first be necessary. Achieving eye contact with the stranger brought the observer somewhat closer to this possibility, but eye contact with alluring people is something that can occur numerous times a day without any clear prospect of further development. With interaction, however, all of this changes. For once strangers "say their first hello," it might well seem that, as the song puts it, "love [that is, making love] was just a glance away, a warm embracing dance away." This is because in face-to-face interaction the two participants are physically close to each other, typically within touching distance. That is, there is no physical barrier to stop the observer, who is under the allure of the stranger, from now reaching out and taking the alluring stranger in a "warm embracing dance," which is just what the allure has been pulling him toward all along. This can easily create an intensified sense of impending physical contact with the other person.

One can also be physically close to an unnoticing or merely contacted stranger. But in these cases the crucial step of interaction has not yet taken place. This step is crucial because once the interaction has commenced, each individual is more or less given tacit permission by the other to continue the interaction. This is also implied by the use of words and phrases such as "Hello," "Hi," "Good morning," and so on, that are typically used to start an interaction. This phatic communication, as it is called, conveys no information. It is merely a way of enabling communication to continue by saying, in effect, "I should like to continue interacting with you." When the other person replies with a similar phatic communication, he or she is replying in effect, "And so should I," or at least leaving this possibility open. Whether and how long the interaction continues will naturally depend on numerous factors. It may simply stop after this exchange. If, however, the interaction does continue, then this too can intensify the stranger's allure. It does so, I would argue, by extending the time during which the observer experiences the intensified sense of impending physical contact with the other person.

With this much said, it might also be felt that the allure of the stranger is intensified if the stranger reciprocates by showing sexual interest in the observer. For this sort of reciprocation definitely can happen, and when it does, it might seem that such an interest coming from the stranger will increase the stranger's sexual attractiveness for the observer. My feeling, however, is that this is not really what happens in such a situation. It is true that we normally like people who like us, but it is not true that we are normally sexually attracted to people who are sexually attracted to us. Similarly, although people's increased liking for us will tend to increase our liking for them, people's increased sexual attraction to us will not tend to increase our sexual attraction to them. This is because, as I argued earlier, sexual attraction is based on physical appearance, and an individual's physical appearance is not affected by the fact that he or she is sexually attracted to another person.

People do, however, change their perception of other people, including their perception of another person's physical appearance. One can, for example, begin to see someone as sexually attractive even though one did not originally find that person to be sexually attractive. And this might not have anything to do with noticing aspects of the person's appearance that were not noticed before. It might simply be that one suddenly sees the person "in a new way," or some such thing. Further, this new way of seeing the person might well be caused by the awareness that the other person finds oneself to be sexually attractive. All of this could be true. My point is merely that there is nothing in the fact that another person finds oneself to be sexually attractive that implies one will therefore find him or her to be sexually attractive. Further, there is no evidence to suggest that there is any connection between the sexual attraction that two people might feel to each other.

This does not mean that someone who feels sexual attraction to another person is sexually unaffected if the other person shows reciprocal sexual attraction. Someone might, for example, decide that the other person's sexual attraction to him suggests that there is a fair chance the other person can be persuaded to see him again or to have sex with him. The person might then, because of the reciprocated attraction, show even more sexual interest in the person and even attempt to realize this goal. This does not mean that the person he is now pursuing with increased vigor has become more sexually attractive. It only means that the reciprocated sexual attraction has encouraged him to pursue the other person sexually. It is easy to understand how someone might misinterpret this state of affairs to mean that the other person's sexual attraction to him has increased his own sexual attraction to her. I think, however, a careful observation of the situation will show that this is typically not what happens.

I mentioned that with the advent of interaction with a stranger, all sorts of other possibilities suggest themselves. One such possibility is the loss of the stranger's strangerness. That is, as I showed in the previous section, a stranger whom one is interacting with is in the process of quickly losing his or her status as a stranger. If the interaction is brief with little exchange of information—either verbal or nonverbal—then the stranger remains more or less a stranger. If, on the other hand, the interaction continues for 5 to 10 minutes with a clear exchange of information, then the person interacting with the stranger will see the person's status as a stranger slowly changing into that of an acquaintance. In the case of an alluring stranger, this means that an alluring stranger becomes an alluring acquaintance and, depending on the nature of the interaction, perhaps becomes even an alluring friend. This alters the context of the allure in a dramatic way. Just how this works will be the subject of the next chapter. There remains, however, another aspect of strangers and allure that should first be dealt with.

STRANGERS IN DREAMS

I said earlier that there is a sense in which all strangers are strangers in the night. This is because just as things in the night are partially hidden from view, so are strangers. There are, however, other strangers, or rather representations of strangers, who are literally, and always, strangers in the night. These are the strangers we meet among the characters in our dreams. Strangers are, in fact, quite common in dreams. According to some reports, about 50 per cent of dream character are strangers, while in some individuals' series of dreams, 80 percent of the characters can be strangers.[17] Also attending dreams are romantic partners, who appear on average in about 20 percent of dreams,[18] and core family members (mother, father, and siblings), who tend to appear in 10–30 percent of dreams.[19]

It is understandable that lovers and core family members appear in our dreams, for these are usually the significant persons in our lives. And it seems reasonable to suppose that we would commonly dream about people who are significant to us. This much, at least, follows from the continuity hypothesis about dreaming.[20] According to this hypothesis, dreams have a continuity with our waking lives. In other words, things that are significant to us in our waking lives reappear in varied forms in our dreams. But why, then, should strangers make such a prominent appearance? Since strangers are unknown people, they seem to lack much of what would make them significant. And in lacking significance in our waking lives, there seems little reason to dream about them.

One way to approach this question would be to ask whether strangers really do lack significance. As I have argued throughout this chapter, an alluring stranger can have a strong effect on an observer. This gives such a stranger a powerful significance, if not in the observer's life, then at least in her awareness. Consequently, it makes sense that, on the continuity hypothesis, one might dream about alluring strangers. Of course, this only applies to the alluring stranger, and it might be felt that not all the strangers in our dreams are alluring. Allure cannot thus explain the preponderance of strangers in our dreams.

The problem, however, is that dream strangers, like many dream characters or even other dream elements, are not always what they seem. This distinction between what a dream element is and what it seems to be is a distinction made by Freud in his theory of dream interpretation.[21] The images we encounter in our dreams are what Freud calls the manifest dream content. This manifest content, however, is a symbolic representation of other hidden mental elements, what Freud calls latent dream thoughts. Consequently, in this view, although a dream image or character might appear to be one thing, it is usually symbolic for another. The reason for this transformation of the latent dream thought into the manifest dream content is because the dream thoughts often display an unconscious desire that the dreamer would find disturbing or repulsive. Changing them into disguised or symbolic dream images is a way of expressing or satisfying the desire while still keeping it hidden. In this view, strangers in dreams might not be strangers at all but rather people we know, people whom the dream work has transformed into strangers in order to keep their identities hidden.

An important mechanism by which such identities are hidden is well known to anyone who has examined his or her dreams. This is the mechanism by which various related images are merged together into one composite, a process that is called condensation. A careful look at strangers in dreams will reveal that they are often not complete strangers but are rather a blend of various people we know. When I have listened to people describe their dreams and have pressed them to say a bit more about a stranger who appears in the dream, it is frequently the case that they can discern various features of other people who have been blended in with the stranger.

Sometimes these features come from several people, sometimes from only a few.

Evidence for the view that strangers in dreams are often known dream characters who have been transformed into unknown strangers is found in a major study by dream researcher Calvin Hall.[22] Hall collected nearly 3,000 dreams from over 2,000 subjects in order to test an aspect of the Oedipal complex. In the last chapter I discussed that aspect of the Oedipal complex that refers to children's tendency to be sexually attracted to their opposite-sex parent and, consequently, later in life to be sexually attracted to persons who resemble their opposite-sex parent. Another part of the Oedipal complex is that because very young children are strongly attracted and attached to their mother, they tend to see the father as an intruding stranger who threatens to take the mother away. (Little girls later shift their attraction from the mother to the father.)

Basing his ideas on this account, and also on the continuity hypothesis of dreaming, Hall came up with several hypotheses about the appearances of strangers in dreams. Three central hypotheses are, first, that the dreamer would have a greater number of aggressive encounters with male strangers than with female strangers, familiar males, or familiar females. A further hypothesis is that the number of aggressive encounters with male strangers would be greater for male dreamers than for female dreamers (since females have a more ambivalent relationship with their fathers). The final central hypothesis was that when asked to free associate with the male strangers in the dream (that is, to say what comes to one's mind first when one thinks of the male dream stranger), subjects in the study would think of either their father or male authority figures. Free association is a technique that can be used to uncover the latent dream thoughts that lie behind the manifest content. In using free association, the person who had the dream merely reflects on a particular element in the dream and says the first thing that comes to his or her mind. Since the manifest dream content is a symbolic representation of the latent dream thought, it is likely that an unguarded or free association to the manifest dream element will reveal what the element symbolizes.

An analysis of the dream contents along with the use of free association with the subjects confirmed each of these hypotheses. This supports the idea that male strangers in dreams tend to be or to represent the dreamer's father. The most powerful support for this seems to come from the results of the free association. For the fact that the subjects in the study immediately tended to think of their fathers or male authority figures does suggest that the male strangers were symbolic expression of their fathers. Of course, a male authority figures does not necessarily represent one's father, but the symbolic relation between the idea of a male authority figure and a father seems strong enough to suggest a connection here, especially since these were the two major associations given by the subjects.

Now, although this study does not examine the presence or meaning of alluring strangers who appear in dreams, it does show how such dream characters can have a fairly common hidden identity. It also shows how such an identity can be traced back to an element of the Oedipal complex. This immediately raises the question of whether alluring dream strangers also symbolize an element of the Oedipal complex, namely, the sexually attractive opposite-sex parent. As I suggested in the last chapter, there is evidence that the experience of allure often has its roots in childhood sexual attraction to the opposite-sex parent. If this is true, and if it is true that aggressive male strangers in dreams tend to represent the dreamer's father, then it seems reasonable to suppose that alluring male strangers in women's dreams might represent the dreamer's father while alluring females in men's dreams might represent the dreamer's mother.

But why should these parental figures appear as strangers in the dream? By Hall's account, the reason the father appears as a stranger in the dream is that, as a young child, the dreamer experienced him as an intrusive stranger. Although Hall's research primarily focused on the appearance of the father as an aggressive stranger, it is easily understandable how, for the female dreamer, the father could also appear as an alluring stranger. For once the father has been symbolized as an aggressive stranger, the associative connection between father and stranger has already been formed. Consequently, when the father later takes on a sexual attractiveness for the little girl, his later representation in her dreams simply shifts from an aggressive stranger to an alluring stranger or even remains aggressive while at the same time becoming alluring. There might also be other reasons for the alluring father's taking on the guise of a stranger in a woman's dream. As stated in Chapter One, for some people feelings of guilt, shame, or revulsion can result from the awareness of a sexual attraction to his or her opposite-sex parent. Disguising the alluring parental dream character as a stranger would be one way of hiding this attraction from oneself.

Still, none of this means that the alluring stranger in a woman's dream need also be aggressive. It only shows that, because of the Oedipal origins of the male dream stranger, for the woman dreamer there can be a relation between the aggressive and alluring male dream stranger. To explore these ideas, let us now look at some dreams where these themes appear. I should say, however, that the dreams I have chosen come from a large collection of dreams that have been brought together by dream researchers Adam Schneider and G. William Domhoff.[23] I have therefore not had a chance to discuss any of the dreams with the subjects (and some of the subjects are anonymous anyway). This means that any interpretation I give can only be very tentative. Nevertheless, there are several themes in these dreams that point to an understanding of alluring dream strangers. To start, let us see how a woman's idea of her father and an alluring dream stranger can be related by looking at the following section of a dream. The dreamer is a woman in her 50s:

> I now am walking back to my home and I see a vast ocean, a beautiful blue color. The color is quite special and I am entranced by it. I see a whale fluking his tail (tale [*sic*]) and then feeding right at the line where the gray shallow water and the blue deep water meet. I feel intense joy at the privilege of seeing this beauty. I am so drawn to it that I feel pulled like a lemming to swim out in it and drown—suicide, drown myself under the blue water, being swallowed by the whale. It's scary. Suddenly I turn and realize there is a man standing right behind me, ready to stop me if I choose to jump into the ocean. I notice his eyes are exactly the same shade of blue as the ocean. I am totally drawn to him. We sit and talk. He says, "Let's get married." I hesitate. We're strangers, but I know he's the one I trust. I say yes.[24]

There are several themes in this dream, and it impossible to say precisely what they signify without discussing the dream with the dreamer. It is, however, clear that there is a male stranger in the dream to whom the dreamer is strongly attracted (the strength of the attraction, along with the fact that he asks to marry her, suggests it is sexual attraction). The strength of her attraction to him is partly expressed, it seems, by the connection she notices between the stranger and the beautiful blue color of the vast ocean. For when she turns to see the stranger what she notices about his appearance is that his eyes are exactly the same beautiful shade of blue. And just as she is drawn to the ocean—she says, "I am so drawn to it that I feel pulled like a lemming to swim out in it and drown"—so is she "totally drawn" to the stranger with the blue eyes. Her feeling pulled to swim out and drown herself under the beautiful blue water, and be swallowed by a whale sounds much like her feeling pulled toward the stranger. Her too she could feel pulled to swim into and drown in the blue of his eyes, so to speak, being swallowed up by him like a whale. And to a little girl her father might well appear to be as vast as an ocean and huge as a whale. Being swallowed by him might even assure her that she had, as the advertisement in the last chapter put it, "skin good enough to eat" and that he was therefore drawn to her even as she was allured to him.

Further, it is apparent that the stranger takes a protective and thus fatherly role toward the dreamer. He is, for example, standing behind the dreamer and ready to stop her if she tries to jump in the water, much like a father watching protectively over his daughter at the beach.

Another thing that points to the fatherly identity of the stranger is his saying to the dreamer, "Let's get married." The fact that he says it without any obvious lead-up to such a proposal does not make it sound like something an adult man would say to adult woman. Rather, it sounds like something a father would say playfully to his small daughter. As is well known, many little girls of four or five will say to their fathers, "When I grow up, Daddy, I'm going to marry you." The father's playful reply could easily be, "Yes, let's get married." Or, on another occasion, seeing the joy in her eyes when she smiles at him, he could show how special she is by saying, "Let's get married!"

A further element that makes the character seem like her father is that the dreamer says, "I know he's the one I trust," and then agrees to marry him. But how can she know she can trust a complete stranger she has just met? A possible answer is that he is only a stranger at the level of the manifest dream content. At the level of the latent dream thought, he is her father. This is why the dreamer knows she can trust him and also agrees to marry him (just as she, as a little girl, might quickly agree when her father says to her, "Let's get married"). Yet it is nevertheless confusing for her; for even though she is somehow aware that the dream character is her father, she also experiences him as a stranger. It is almost as if she is taken in by the disguise but at the same time is vaguely aware of his real identity. This is why she hesitates.

Let us now look at a young man's dream of an attractive unknown woman:

> This dream, as I recall it, begins earlier, but I remember it begins at a very elite party, very uppercrust, and for what reason, I have no idea, but I'm there. I believe everyone is dressed in tuxedos and evening gowns, and the instant that I clearly remember began when a most complex piece of design that was decorating the place is some way centrally involved with the activity of the evening, made out of cardboard or silvered (antepaper?) [*sic*] became disarrayed, and I think it was supposed to be my fault or something, but at any rate, I attempted to strike [straighten?] it out. The next thing I remember I was in a

> hallway and two women were helping me straighten it out, either one was on an end of it and that made them approximately 12 ft. away from one another, and I was underneath trying to straighten this rather complex design. I would sort of crawl on the floor from one to the other, trying to straighten it out because it seemed to be the only way. I became somewhat enamored with one of the women, even though both of their skirts were rather tight around their knees, the one that I thought was also slightly interested in me, I may have kissed her on the calf and I believe she liked it and sort of presented her other calf to be kissed, which I think I did. Then just out of sheer devilishness, I crept back, fixing the design and kissed the other one on the calf, which didn't go over too big. As a matter of fact, I was quite certain that she was shocked and was possibly indignant about it, but I just chuckled to myself and continued about my work. The rather curvaceous and attractive woman at the other end was moving about and I caressed her legs again and put my hands on and then finally I think I got this complex design straightened out.[25]

Again, without hearing the man's associations to this dream, the full significance of the various elements cannot be known. Nevertheless, there are several elements in the dream that suggest that the curvaceous and attractive stranger he becomes enamored with might represent his own mother. This is indicated first by the infantile role the man plays in his dream, which points to the idea that his sexual attraction to the woman is a representation of his sexual attraction as a child to his own mother. First, it is noteworthy that the dream starts off with the dreamer finding himself at a party with no idea why he is there. This sounds much like a small child's awareness of being brought to a party or gathering, as small children often are, but having no awareness of what the purpose of the party is or why he should be brought to it. Secondly, there is a central activity going on that he does not understand, just as a toddler might observe an event at an adult's party with no understanding of the point behind the activity. Thirdly, just as a toddler at such a function might make a mess or cause a disarray while being vaguely aware that he is responsible, so also is the dreamer aware that the disarray is somehow supposed to be his fault.

An example of such an event that the dreamer is describing could be a Christmas gathering where people are decorating a Christmas tree, which could be the central activity of the evening. The cardboard and silvered paper could be the decorations. The disarray could then be when the small child pulled at the decorations, causing the tree to fall over.

The fourth thing that makes the man look like he has an infantile role in the dream is that he finds himself crawling on the floor back and forth between two women. This looks very much like the behavior of a small child crawling playfully back and forth between his mother and another woman. Fifthly, although he seems to be trying to fix the problem that he is aware of having caused, he is also, like a small child, being mischievous at the same time.

The nearby woman he is enamored with would appear to be his mother. This is because whenever an infant is crawling about, its mother—the woman the infant is typically enamored with—is usually nearby. That she is his mother is supported by the fact that he kisses her calf, that she likes it, that she presents the other calf to be kissed, and that he later caresses and puts his hands on her legs. This seems much like mother-child interaction. There is another woman nearby, but she has a very different relation to the dreamer. When he kisses her leg, he does it out of "sheer devilishness," not because he is enamored with her or because she is curvaceous and attractive. Further, she herself does not like it, does not present the other leg, and becomes indignant.

An obvious critique of the interpretations I have given for the two dreams is to claim that nothing in the dream descriptions indicates definitely that the alluring stranger represents the dreamer's opposite-sex parent. Further, it might be claimed that with enough ingenuity, any dream could be interpreted in such a way as to show that an alluring stranger symbolizes the male or female dreamer's opposite-sex parent.

My reply to these points is that I agree. Nevertheless, it remains true that some dreams containing alluring strangers are more suggestive of the interpretation I have been giving than others are. Consider the following dream by a woman:

> I keep seeing this guy around—he's pretty good-looking, seems nice, not flashy or even very outgoing, probably younger than me—we go to the same school or work in the same place, I'm not sure—I notice him a lot but I don't ever speak, we haven't actually met and now he's sitting next to me in a movie theater. I'm with some other people but I'm pretty distracted by him. I think he's with other people too but not with a girl. I get more agitated as time goes on, and very late in the movie he turns his head toward me, leans over very slowly and kisses me. Suddenly I know he's noticed me too, and is as attracted to me as I am to him. I'm shocked, but I turn my head to him and kiss him back, on the lips. I really want him. My feelings are very strong.[26]

Plainly, nothing in this dream suggests that the distracting stranger symbolizes the dreamer's father. Rather, he is simply a "good-looking" man who she kisses at the cinema and who she feels strongly for. This is quite different from the first two dreams I looked at. In those dreams it was not too difficult to discern elements that tied the alluring stranger to the dreamers' opposite-sex parent. This does not mean, however, that the kissing stranger in the dream just given does not symbolize the dreamer's father. For it might well be that this stranger's tie to the dreamer's father is simply better hidden than in the previous two dreams. If and why this is the case is something that could only be explored through a discussion with the woman or through her free associations.

It is important to remember, however, that there are general considerations that can suggest a common interpretation of particular dream content. Hall's research, for example, suggested that aggressive male strangers in dreams tend to symbolize the dreamer's father. There are also, as I argued, general considerations that indicate that, for the female dreamer, the alluring male stranger will tend to represent her father. In addition, there is, I would argue, a general consideration that indicates that, for both the male and female dreamer, an alluring female stranger will tend to represent the dreamer's mother. There are, of course, the common negative feelings mentioned earlier that often seem associated with this idea. These might lead to the dream thought of one's mother being transformed into the character of an alluring stranger. But there is a more basic and universal consideration that needs to be mentioned. This is the existential fact that we are all born into a world of strangers and, further, that the first stranger who significantly deals with us will tend to be our mother. She is also our first real encounter with a person. She is thus the prototypical stranger: the stranger who precedes all other strangers. In addition to this, she is also an alluring stranger: the warmth of her skin, the softness of her breasts, and the succulence of her smell would all seem to combine in the infant's awareness to draw the infant magnetically toward her. Because of this she is also the prototype of an alluring stranger. There is thus a sense in which all subsequent alluring female strangers are, in our awareness, a copy of her.

It is natural to wonder here just how much of the mother's warmth, softness, and succulence a newborn infant is aware of. And, indeed, not too many years ago the accepted view was that the neonate has no real awareness of its environment and the people within it. In 1967, for example, Benjamin Spock told the world that up to two or three months of age, the infant has little contact with external things, focusing instead on its own physical states.[27] Now, however, there is good evidence to suggest that shortly after birth the infant is able to discern things in its surroundings and even maintain eye contact.[28] In the first 45 minutes after birth, an infant will typically maintain a state of high alertness while it visually attends to the various events and objects in its environment. One prominent object is its mother.

One issue that needs to be addressed here is the problem of the difference between the male and female situation. For if the mother is also alluring for the female infant, why then does the female typically go on to find males rather than females alluring? (For as I argue in the last chapter, the experience of allure seems to have its origins in the allure of the opposite-sex parent.) This is a question that has perplexed researchers for a long time, and there is no generally accepted answer. One thing that seems likely, however, is that at some point in the girl's early development, the father typically becomes alluring for her. This might well have something to do with her trying to express independence from the mother. Since the mother is, like herself, a female, turning to her father is a way of expressing her distinctiveness from her mother by attaching herself to someone who, being a male, is distinct from herself. This tie to her father can then easily become eroticized and thus loosen the allure of her mother. Still, because of her early attraction to her mother, this allure never fully disappears. It is for this reason, I would argue, that alluring female strangers can still appear in heterosexual women's dreams and that heterosexual women can still, to some degree, find other women alluring, at least in a way that men tend not to find other men alluring.[29]

With the little boy, things are quite different. Being a male, he is already distinct from the mother, at least in this regard. Consequently, his interest in his father is not, like the girl's, based on an attempt to express distinctiveness from his mother. It is rather an attempt to affiliate to and learn from someone who is like himself. As a result, he typically does not eroticize the tie to his father, and accordingly there is no loosening of the allure of his mother.

Although this account might seem to apply only to the Western nuclear family, it is important to note that even in cultures where child rearing is shared by people outside the immediate family, the mother is still typically the one who spends the most time with the small child.[30] Further, although some cultures have mating systems where women can have sexual intercourse with several men and thus not know who the child's father is (and does not Western culture also partake somewhat of this system?), the important thing for the child's development is not that a biological father is present, but only that there is one or more males—be he the mother's brother, cousin, or close friend—who plays what we would call a father-like role for the little girl.

This would be enough to enable a male to become alluring for her, while at the same time loosening the allure of her mother.

With this we are at last able to arrive at a peculiar conclusion regarding the relation between those individuals whom people find alluring and the alluring strangers they dream of at night. One relation, to be sure, is that both are alluring. The other is that both tend to have symbolic relations to the opposite-sex parent. There is, however, another relation that does not immediately suggest itself but nevertheless seems significant. This is the relation of being strangers. I mentioned earlier that the appearance of dream strangers consists of blended images of different people that form one composite, which in turn renders the character's identity unknown, that is, renders him or her a stranger. But this is very similar to how an alluring person presents herself to the attracted person's awareness. For if an alluring individual tends to resemble the observer's opposite-sex parent, then there is a sense in which such an individual is also seen to be a composite. This is the composite of the observer's image of his or her opposite-sex parent blended with images of some other unknown person or persons. This follows from the fact that the alluring individual is not an exact copy of the observer's opposite-sex parent, but only has a resemblance. Consequently, there are other physical features that make up the alluring person's appearance, features that do not resemble the opposite-sex parent. But these features serve to alter the perception of the person in a peculiar way. For although the familiar features make the observer feel he knows the person, the unfamiliar features work against this feeling to assure him he does not know the person. As a result, the alluring person, even if not a stranger, cannot help but appear to the observer's awareness as something of a stranger.

THREE

Just Friends

FRIENDSHIP

If one of the things a stranger can become is an acquaintance, then one of the things an acquaintance can become is a friend. However, although it may be easy to distinguish a stranger from an acquaintance, it is not always easy to distinguish an acquaintance from a friend, at least in those cases where there is both mutual liking between oneself and one's acquaintance and there are no barriers to friendship.[1] Of course, at one end of the spectrum there are friendly individuals one likes but who are clearly just acquaintances and in no way friends. At the other end there are friends who are plainly more than just acquaintances with whom one has a mutual liking. The problem comes when one tries to find the point at which such an acquaintance becomes a friend. This is a problem, because there can be a person who is both something of an acquaintance and something of a friend. Such an individual may be someone you enjoy seeing and who enjoys seeing you, whom you have met on various occasions, with whom you perhaps have exchanged some personal information, and whom you might even care about. Nevertheless, you do not regularly see each other and are not much involved with each other's life.

It might well be that, as has been suggested, the relation of being an acquaintance can be a barrier to friendship. In this view, rather than being nearly a friendship, an acquaintanceship can be a way of controlling or preventing the warmth and intimacy of friendship. This is plainly true in some instances. In such situations the acquaintances have no real liking for each other but merely smile or chat briefly when they meet as a form of ritualistic acknowledgment. But this, it seems to me, is not all that distinct from the way in which interacted-with strangers might treat each other. Further, the preventing of warmth and intimacy is clearly not an element in all acquaintanceships. This is obvious from the fact that in many friendships the friends were first acquaintances. In these cases the acquaintanceship was not a barrier to friendship but a prelude to it.

Because of this lack of clear distinction between friends and acquaintances, my feeling is that if sexual attraction enters into one's relationship with a particular acquaintance, it will tend to be similar to either the sexual attraction felt for an interacted-with stranger or sexual attraction felt toward a friend. Which it is will then depend on whether the acquaintance is more like a stranger or more like a friend. To continue with this inquiry, therefore, it seems appropriate that we turn our eye to the question of sexual attraction in friendship. But what is friendship?

Here it should first be noted that friendship is typically thought of as an interpersonal relationship that does not involve sexual attraction. It may be a close and warm relationship in which two people seek out each other's company, care for each other, and enjoy spending time together, but where the idea of sexual attraction is normally seen as being foreign to the relationship. One obvious reason for this thought is that when people conceive of friendship, they seem to typically have in mind same-sex friendships between heterosexuals. Therefore, the friendship of two heterosexual men or two heterosexual women does not include sexual attraction because in each case the friends belong to the same sex. Sexual attraction for heterosexuals would be something that is normally only experienced toward the opposite sex.

It is true that some scholars have argued that there is an erotic component in most close friendships, even same-sex heterosexual friendships.[2] But this will depend on how exactly one wants to define the idea of "erotic component." In terms of sexual desire and sexual attraction existing within same-sex friendships, I would definitely agree that such components are far more ubiquitous than most people realize. In my view, however, the decisive feature of such components is that they refer to an intimate caressing of naked bodies. If this, then, is how the idea of erotic component is to be understood, then it does not seem obvious that the majority of heterosexual same-sex close relationships have this sort of erotic component. Such a component can, of course, be involved in an apparently heterosexual same-sex relationship since, as I mentioned in the first chapter, homosexuality is not an all-or-nothing affair. This is particularly so when it is realized that people are not always conscious of their own homosexual tendencies. Nevertheless, it seems unlikely that the attraction to the baring and caressing of a same-sex friend is normally present among heterosexual friends.

When one allows the idea, however, that opposite-sex persons can also be friends, not immediately conceiving of friendship as only a same-sex phenomenon, then it becomes obvious that sexual attraction can easily be involved and widely spread. One of the possible reasons why same-sex friendship comes first to mind when someone thinks of friendship is that, until recently, cross-sex friendships were not at all common. In one study from the 1950s, for example, very few people reported having a friend of the opposite sex.[3] This has changed in the last few decades with studies from the United States showing about 40 percent of men and 30 percent of women having at least one cross-sex friend.[4] One recent study from Greece found that 80 percent of those studied had or previously had close cross-sex friends.

This indicates that the situation has dramatically changed in recent times or at least has done so in Western culture, where people have freedom to choose their friends. In many countries with oppressive regimes or in cultures driven by religious fundamentalism, men and women who are not married to each other are often not even allowed to be alone together. In these cultures there is no possibility for cross-sex friendship.

There are also other cultures where although it is not illegal or religiously disallowed for unmarried men and women to be friends, it is nevertheless socially criticized to the point where few would dare to have a cross-sex friend. A 29-year-old woman from Beijing whom I interviewed assured me that even in the Chinese capital, adult cross-sex friendships are rarely found. If a young man and woman are regularly seen together, she said, people will expect them to be either dating, engaged, or married. If they are not and are merely friends, their peers would be highly critical of the situation, and their parents might simply step in and demand the termination of the friendship. Also, if a married man or woman attempted to have a cross-sex friend, the spouse would never allow it.

The one possible exception, she told me, was in the case of couple friendships, that is, friendships between one dating or married couple and another. Here, when the two couples meet, an individual from one couple would be allowed to chat and show friendly behavior toward the opposite-sex individual from the other couple, but only in the presence of the other members of the foursome. Further, the principal friendships within such couple friendships would be between the same-sex individuals, with the men showing their friendship mainly to each other and the women showing their friendship mainly to each other (evidence suggests this pattern is also true of Western couple friendships). The cross-sex friendships in these couple friendships would never be close or intimate. Oddly enough, although many Chinese wives would bitterly complain if their husband had a woman friend, they frequently accept that their husband might have several mistresses. Although one might assume that this would be because the relationship to the mistress would be kept from public view, even a furtive friendship with a woman, she told me, would be severely opposed by the wife. In this culture, too, there seems little possibility for cross-sex friendships.

Nevertheless, even within contemporary Western culture and its growing number of cross-sex friendships, it still seems that cross-sex friendships are viewed with misgiving. The reason for this is probably related to the fact that the majority of people still prefer same-sex friendships. Consequently, such people might well think that if someone has a cross-sex friend, it must be for reasons other than friendship. In this view, cross-sex friendships are seen as essentially a preliminary to a romantic or at least a sexual relationship. The underlying idea here seems to be that men and women cannot be just friends, or at least that the idea of friendship, so far as it is just a friendship, cannot involve a sexual relationship or even sexual attraction.

This idea is expressed in many popular films from the 1980s and onward, such as *When Harry Met Sally*, *Boys and Girls*, and *My Best Friend's Wedding*. In these and other films the story usually involves a single man and woman who are friends. Although they are not sexually involved, they spend time with each other as their lives take various twists and turns. In the end they finally fall in love, or at least one of them does, or perhaps they first have sex and then fall in love. In this way such films support the belief that women and men cannot be friends without it leading to a sexual relationship. The notion that cross-sex friendships are but a prelude to love in turn seems founded on the more basic idea that sexual attraction must play a role in cross-sex friendships. To see where this idea comes from, let us start by examining the idea of friendship itself.

Probably the earliest and best-known account of the nature of friendship is given by Aristotle, a keen observer of humanity. According to his account, friendship is an interpersonal relationship based on mutual liking. Liking toward anyone, he tells us, means "wishing for him what you believe to be good things, not for your own sake but for his, and being inclined, so far as one can, to bring these things about."[5] When two persons bear this mutual well-wishing and well-doing toward each other for each other's sake, and when they think the other feels the same way, then, says Aristotle, they have friendship.

This account is an important one not only for its insight but also because it shows that friendship is not a modern invention or social construction, as some thinkers have argued. The social philosopher Axel Honneth, for example, claims that what we think of as friendship today only emerged with the writings of the Scottish moral philosophers of the 18th century.[6] Yet Aristotle's account points to what most people today would see as basic features of friendship, namely, reciprocity, well-wishing, well-doing, and an awareness of each other's feeling in this regard. Because this ancient view captures the core elements of our modern idea of friendship, it seems that friendship is not, in any deep sense, a modern invention. This does not mean that Aristotle's view fully explains all instances of friendship. Aristotle's account, for example, implies the idea of autonomy where a person freely chooses to treat his or her friend in various ways for the friend's sake. However, in non-Western subsistence economies where people depend strongly on each other for the basics of life, friendships can entail more obligations whereby the exchange of instrumental and material gain are an explicit part of the relationship.[7]

Further, as I mentioned in Chapter One, I can have a mild degree of liking for someone whom I see incidentally on various occasions but have no desire to seek out his company afterward. Even if the person has the same feelings toward me, this does not seem to amount to friendship. Here the liking would have to be strong enough to make the persons, all else being equal, want to seek out each other's company.

In addition, it can be questioned whether liking amounts to the same thing as well-wishing and well-doing for the other person's sake. For it seems that I can easily wish someone well for his own sake, and be inclined to do him well, while neither liking nor disliking him. I might, for example, feel that the other person deserves such treatment, even though I have no particular feelings of liking for him. It would be unusual to wish and do someone well for his own sake if one disliked him. But here I am only suggesting that such well-wishing and well-doing do not necessarily imply liking. To like someone as a friend, it seems to me that one must at least enjoy her company simply for the sake of her company. For the idea of liking seems to carry with it the idea of enjoyment of the person's company. When both persons have this enjoyment toward each other, then they have companionship. It is difficult to define companionship, but it would appear to mean, at least in the sense that I want to use it, having enjoyment in being with someone simply for the sake of being with her (as opposed to other affiliative reasons that have nothing to do with the person herself). When both persons have this companionship (which involves enjoyment) added to their mutual well-wishing and well-doing, and when they think the other has a similar enjoyment, then it would seem they have the basis of friendship.

The fundamental role of enjoying the company of one's friend is also expressed in ancient Chinese ideas of friendship. Confucius, for example, remarks, "Is this not delightful that friends should come from distant quarters?"[8] This delight in friends is something that Confucian scholars have pointed to as a basic component of the Confucian, and thus Chinese, concept of friendship.[9] The degree of enjoyment, however, might show some cultural variation. One study, for example, found that American young adults reported higher friendship quality and more happiness in both their same-sex and cross-sex friendships than did Turkish young adults.[10]

Still, what people see as friendships can take many forms. Aristotle himself recognized this when he suggested that there are at least three types of friendships. These were what he called friendship for mutual pleasure, friendship for mutual advantage, and friendship based primarily on the wishing of and doing good for each other. Although most people would probably recognize these types of friendship, there remains a wide range of elements that are also cited as being essential to friendship, with the result that there are many different ideas about what constitutes friendship. Thus, in describing the nature of friendship, people will, in addition to reciprocity, often list such elements as trust, openness, honesty, safety, support, loyalty, constancy, understanding, companionship, shared activities, and acceptance. Many people, however, do not see all of these elements as being essential to any particular friendship. One reason for this is that people seem to want different things out of friendship. For one person, what is important is that a friend is a confidant with whom he or she can be open and honest and feel accepted. For another, what might be essential is that a friend is a loyal companion who likes to do shared activities. Another reason is that, even for one person, different friends address different wants and needs. People are, after all, multifaceted in what they enjoy and what they feel they want out of a friendship. Consequently, what someone sees as being essential to one of his friendships he might not see as being essential to another of his friendships. Or again, while one friendship may satisfy mainly one desire, another friendship may satisfy several desires.

Now, although such a person might enjoy this diversity of friendships and never expect or even want one particular friend to satisfy all his needs, not everyone is like this. Another person might feel that a friend, or at least an ideal friend, is a person who would both value her various aspects and fulfill all of her different requirements. This view of friendship is put forward by a 53-year-old woman in Lillian B. Rubin's study, who says, that

> at the ideal end of the spectrum would be the friend who knows and can value all parts of you. What I mean is, supposing you have ten parts to yourself. With most people you can interact and share maybe one or two of them. Sometimes you get lucky and you can share more than that. And once or twice in a lifetime maybe, with real luck, you find someone you can share all of your ten parts with. Then you only have to hope that, as any of those parts change in yourself, they continue to mesh with the other person. Or, if you're luckiest of all, you'll both keep changing and growing in the same direction.[11]

Such a view of friendship does not exclude the idea that one might nevertheless desire more than one friend. One could simply like the idea of having various friends, each of whom one could share everything with. As this person suggests, however, having several such friends would be unlikely. When one has only one such friend, or rather someone approaching this idealized sort of friend, then this approaches the idea of a "best friend." For one of the important features of a best friend appears to be the ability, as this woman puts it, to "continue to mesh with the other person." This is because "best friendship" looks like it requires an ability to persist through various changes in a way that other forms of friendship might not. Therefore, to call someone one's best friend is at the same time to say, among other things, that he or she has been one's friend for an extended period of time. Although it would be acceptable to call someone a friend whom one only met a few weeks ago, it would typically not do to call such a person one's best friend. And if a friendship is one that persists through an extended period of time, then it must be a friendship that can adjust itself to the various changes both of the parties will most likely go through. Perhaps the friendship starts when both persons are single. But then one of them finds a partner or gets married. This change of life circumstances for one of the friends will often put a stress on the friendship, with, say, the married friend spending more time with his or her spouse or, as is often the case, with the spouse feeling threatened by the old friendship or even trying to terminate the friendship.

This is not to say that a best friendship will necessarily survive this sort of pressure while a non-best friendship will not. For, of course, many best friendships draw to a close under these or similar life changes. Best friendship would seem, however, to refer to a sort of friendship that would be more flexible and thus more enduring than other forms of friendship.

In addition to the different views about what constitutes friendship, there are also the different contexts in which friendships actually occur. As a result, the elements that might suit a friendship in one context might not suit a friendship in another. For example, the context of the friendship that the woman just cited has in mind would be one in which the two persons were able to keep in regular contact over an extended period of time.

But what about a context in which this was unlikely to happen, a context in which two people meet, become friends, and then part, never to see each other again? Such a friendship can occur when two people meet each other while traveling. For example, on different occasions I have traveled on my own through such places as India, China, and South-East Asia. One of the enjoyable features of such travel is the other independent travelers one continually meets. Therefore, even though I set out to travel on my own, I was hardly ever traveling alone. Arriving at a guest house or an eating place in a particular village, I would often meet another traveler, usually a Westerner, sometimes a male, sometimes a female, sometimes couples, or even groups of three or four. We would share stories about where we had been, difficulties we had encountered and how we had solved them, travel plans, and other information about ourselves. Many times this would lead to a mutual liking and an agreement to travel further together. As the journey continued, these "friendships of the moment," as they could be called, would frequently deepen as we faced together the trials and tribulations of backpacking in, say, a distant corner of India.

Although these friendships would have much to do with the shared activity of traveling, this was hardly the only or even main feature of the relationship. For much time would often be spent in discussion, sharing of ideas and personal feelings, humor, and the enjoyment of each other's company.

Then, however, would come the moment when we parted ways: my companion wanting to head, say, north to Srinagar and I wanting to head, say, south to Kerala. There was often a tinge of sadness in our goodbyes, and sometimes we exchanged contact information. But at the same time, there was usually an acceptance that these were friendships of the moment, that he or she lived on one side of the world and I on another and, consequently, that we would most likely not see each other again. Yet, for all that, some of these relationships were clearly friendships, sharing many of the core features of friendships in other contexts.

Besides the different views of friendship and the different contexts, there are also the factors of age and gender. For example, the friendships of early childhood tend to be based on shared activities or play. In the earliest sort of play, known as parallel play, two or more toddlers simply carry out their activities in close proximity but without interacting. Later there occurs a sort of activity known as sociodramatic play. Children engaged in this will cooperate by pretending and acting out a story they have made up. By middle childhood, however, children's friendships become more psychological, with children tending to value psychological aspects of their friends.[12]

The role of gender in friendship makes its appearance already in early childhood, with the majority of children preferring same-sex friends. This preference is shown by as early as 33 months of age,[13] is something that happens across different cultures,[14] and becomes stronger up until middle childhood.[15]

Not only is this gender segregation a dominant feature in children's friendships, but the features of boys' same-sex friendships seem to differ from that of girls' same-sex friendships. Therefore, in contrast to boys, girls tend to have friendships with one or two friends, have more social conversation, and engage in cooperative play or games that involve turn-taking. Boys, on the other hand, tend to have groups of friends and partake in rough and tumble play and competitive games.[16] Although girls will also spend time in a group, they usually see such a group as a network of two-person intimate relationships. This contrasts with the boys' view that their group is more of a collective entity.[17]

Not all research, however, is consistent on these points. Some studies have found that boys say they have about the same number of friends as girls say they have and, also, that both boys and girls describe their friendships as intimate.[18] Further, this should not be taken to mean that boys do not interact in pairs, for boys interact in pairs just as frequently as girls do. Their dyadic interactions, however, are more short-lived than those of girls.[19] On the other hand, girls' friendships are more fragile and do not seem to last as long as boys' friendships.[20]

By adolescence the tendency for girls to have more intimate friendships than boys seems well established. Adolescent girls' same-sex friendships have more self-disclosure and involve more intimate displays of affection than boys' friendships do. Further, while girls use their friendships in adolescence to help establish their developing sense of becoming sexual adults, boys use their friendships to help gain independence from their families.[21]

By the time of adulthood, it is clear that there are some important differences between the majority of male same-sex friendships and the majority female same-sex friendships. First of all, the evidence suggests that men tend to have fewer friends than women do, with some studies showing that many men have no friends. One study also found that although the majority of women reported having a best friend, over two-thirds of single men were unable to name a best friend. Moreover, as men get older, they tend to lose friends without replacing them. This is quite different from women, who tend to be concerned about having friends and who easily make new friends if they lose old friends. Interestingly, the men who are in these friendless situations appear not to be particularly bothered by it, often claiming that with family and work there is no time left for friends.

Comparing the content of male friendships to female friendships, male friendships tend to have less of an emotional component than do female friendships. Some people have used the word "bonding" to refer to the emotional ties in a male friendship that lack the intensity and intimacy of emotional ties between female friends. Male friendships also tend to be based on shared experiences or activities more than female friendships are. Therefore, when questioned about what they do with their men friends, men tend to report shared activities such as sports, watching sports, or outdoor activities. Further, these activities or shared experiences seem to be basic to the relationship, with little time spent in self-disclosure, intimate discussions of their personal lives, or even any discussion. This feature of male friendships is captured in the story of two men who regularly met at a bar in order to have a drink together (a shared activity). One day, after sitting in the bar for two hours without exchanging a word, one man asks the other, "Do you know what time it is?" The other man replies, "Did we come here to drink or did we come here to talk?"

This is in strong contrast to female friendships, where the relationship typically involves more intense and intimate emotional ties, mutual self-disclosure, emotional support, and the sharing of personal information. Although female friendships can also involve shared activities, it seems it is the intimate exchange of personal information that is the basis of the friendship rather than the activity. Because of these basic differences in men's and women's friendships, which are traceable to the same-sex friendships of early childhood, cross-sex friendships will clearly offer both men and women something distinct from their same-sex friendships.

Before, however, I turn specifically to cross-sex friendships, it seems important to consider the question of why we seek out friends at all. In other words, what is it that lies at the basis of our urge to form friendships?

One answer that has been put forward here is that the human mind is biologically constructed to bond with others.[22] In other words, we are somehow genetically programmed to seek out friends. But this sort of explanation leaves one with the feeling that nothing has really been explained. For such an account implies that the desire to have friends somehow springs into consciousness from nonconscious biological sources. From this view it would seem to follow that when we examine our experience of the desire to have friends, we can give no conscious account of where this desire comes from. Yet it seems clear that we can give reasons why we seek out friends.

Another answer, one given by psychotherapist Lillian B. Rubin, is that the desire for friends originates from a desire to recreate the experience of infancy when we had a special and intimate relationship with our mother or primary caregiver.[23] Although this answer is better in that it at least points to experience for the basis for this conscious desire, it still suffers for other reasons. First, as I have argued elsewhere, there is good evidence that sexual desire, and thus romantic love, has its beginnings in the mother-infant relationship. Also, as I showed in the first chapter of this book, the allure of sexual attraction itself can be traced back to this early relationship or, in the case of the female, also to the early father–daughter relationship.

Now, since the early infant–parent relationship typically involves an intimate and warm baring and caressing of naked skin, especially in breast-feeding, changing, and bathing, but also in kissing, snuggling, stroking, and hugging, then it is understandable that a person leaving his or her childhood behind typically seeks to recreate this intimate skin-to-skin contact.[24] This is the fundamental reason why people seek out sexual interaction, often with a partner who resembles their opposite-sex parent. But if the desire for friendship has this same origin, then it seems it should also be composed of the desires for intimate baring and caressing with one's friend. But it seems obvious that the majority of heterosexual same-sex friendships lack this sexual component, by which I mean a desire for or attraction to a mutual baring and caressing of naked skin (I will come to a discussion of this component in cross-sex friendships in the next section). It *can* occur together with these desires, but such desires are not a core component of friendship, not in the way that they are core components of sexual desire. In other words, if sexual desire or attraction occurs in friendship, it occurs in addition to friendship. Further, it seems unlikely that a person's same-sex friends will tend to resemble his or her opposite-sex parent.

These considerations suggest that the desire for friendship is a somewhat distinct phenomenon from sexual desire and thus has a distinct origin. What, then, is this origin? The answer that I should like to suggest is that we seek out friends because they free us from a deep-rooted metaphysical sense of isolation. What I mean by this sense of isolation is the experience we all have of the complete inaccessibility of another person's mind or consciousness. His or her consciousness seems to exist forever beyond our grasp, undergoing its experiences in a realm we can never enter.

In philosophy this is the basis for what is known as the problem of other minds. This problem springs from the idea that although you might believe that other people have minds with consciousness, ideas, and feelings, there is no way you could ever know this for certain. This is because although you are directly aware of your own consciousness, all you are ever directly aware of with other people is their behavior. You never directly experience their thoughts, ideas, or feelings. Perhaps you are the only conscious being in existence. You might assume other people have minds just like you have a mind, but how can you ever know this is a plausible assumption?

To get an idea of what it would be like to be mistaken about this, think of the characters you meet in your dreams. When you encounter them, they seem like real people with their own minds. They discuss things with you, surprise you with their words and actions, ignore you, show affection toward you, or chase after you. They seem like completely autonomous individuals endowed with their own will, their own ideas, and their own consciousness. But they are not. They are merely dream images that you yourself have thought up. Consequently, even though while you are dreaming, you think they have their own consciousness, you are wrong. But if you can be wrong about the characters you meet in your dreams, then maybe you can be wrong about the people you meet when you are awake. Of course, the people you meet when you are awake are not dream characters (or are they?), but one does not have to be a dream character to lack consciousness while only appearing to have it. There are numerous other ways this could be imagined. How do you know, for example, that other people are not just sophisticated biological organisms, organisms that respond in complex verbal and nonverbal ways, but with no consciousness at all?

The answer is you cannot. This is because the consciousness of another person is something you can never be directly aware of. And this would remain true even if telepathy were possible. For even if you received thoughts that you believed were the thoughts of another person, there is again no way you could check to see if this was true. Even if the "transmitting" person were to confirm that she had sent you the thoughts, this confirmation could only be in the form of verbal or nonverbal behavior. As a result, you could never know if the thought you believed to be telepathically sent was the actual thought of another person. Maybe it was just an electrical impulse sent from the other person's brain, an impulse that caused your own thought.

The view that you are the only consciousness in the world is known as solipsism. And much of the work in the philosophy of knowledge is to try to find a way around solipsism, that is, to find out how we can legitimately claim to know that other minds exist. The desire to solve this problem, I would argue, also springs from the deep-rooted metaphysical sense of isolation. It is, however, a logical response to the sense of isolation, whereas the seeking of friends is an existential response.

To this someone might reply that even if we cannot know for certain that other people have consciousness, it is at least likely that they do. But this reply does not avoid the philosophical problem, for how could we know if it is likely? The only way that we could know this is if there were some way we could test to see if it is. But once again, the inaccessibility of other consciousnesses guarantees that no such test is possible.

Although this might seem like a complex theoretical problem that has little to do with most people's daily lives, I think it is rather a problem that most of us are, at some level, aware of. We are all aware, for example, that our thoughts are our own private territory, learning very early in life that no one but ourselves has direct access to them. It is this knowledge that gives rise, for example, to the common practice of lying. Knowing this, it is natural to infer that, if other persons are like me, then they, too, have a private territory of thoughts that I can never directly enter.

But once one has arrived at this idea, it is but a small step to the next idea, namely: "But if their thoughts are so completely private, how can I even know they have thoughts?" Ideas like this can be disturbing, for they carry with them a sense of being metaphysically isolated. This sort of isolation is, though related, different from that of feeling isolated from other people, people whose existences are, at one level, taken for granted. It is rather an isolation whereby one feels it is entirely possible that there are no other people at all, at least not people with consciousness. This is why I call it metaphysical isolation, for metaphysics refers to the ultimate constituents of reality and, in such a view of reality, the only constituent that is conscious is oneself.

Because such thoughts can be unnerving, they are often swept out of awareness or repressed. But this does not mean they are gone from the mind. We know from psychoanalytic investigations that disturbing thoughts rarely disappear. Rather they are merely repressed or relegated to an unconscious level from which they continue to affect our conscious thoughts and behavior.

One of the effects of such thoughts and the resulting sense of isolation, I would argue, is the search for friends. A prominent result of having a friend is that there is another individual you come to like and know well, someone whose thoughts, ideas, and feelings you deeply understand, empathize with, and nearly sense as your own. This is the idea behind the assertion of the Roman philosopher Cicero that "a friend is, as it were, another self."[25] Further, as a friend, the other person has the same experience of you.

In achieving this closeness one gains a sense of acquiring direct access to another mind, of directly revealing one's own mind to another mind, and thus a sense of shedding one's metaphysical isolation. One can, to be sure, know well someone who is not one's friend or even someone whom one dislikes. But in this case the sense that one has of the person lacks the closeness and warmth that one experiences in the mutual liking with a friend. And it is this closeness and warmth, along with the intimate knowledge of the other person, that works to create the sensation of having some sort of access the other person's mind. Because of the enjoyment involved in being with one's friend, the ideas and feelings that the friend expresses can take on a warm and familiar quality that makes them seem nonforeign and easily accessible. Yet even here one does not really gain direct access to the mind of another, which is why Cicero must qualify his claim with "as it were." Nevertheless, what friendship does is to bring us as close as possible experientially to solving the problem of other minds, thus weakening our sense of metaphysical isolation. And herein lies its fundamental motive, though, of course, several other motives can accompany it.

A possible objection to this view might be to argue that such ponderings are far too complicated for small children to entertain. Yet, the argument could continue, small children also seek out friends. Therefore, the conclusion could be that the desire to avoid metaphysical isolation cannot be the basic motive for friendship.

There are, however, various replies that could be made to this. First, I agree that small children, at least under the age of five, do not normally entertain the idea of metaphysical isolation. Indeed, even within the first year of life they already employ what is called a "theory of mind," that is, the attributing of mental states to other persons in order to explain their behavior. Still, by as early as three years of age, most children are capable of lying. This suggests that a child of this early age has already acquired at least a minimal awareness of the idea that his or her own mind is inaccessible to other people. For lying only makes sense if the person lying believes that the person he is lying to has no direct access to his or her thoughts. Normally the child will not see the implications of this idea—that other people's minds are likewise inaccessible to him—but the seeds for this realization are already sown.

Further, the friendships of this early age are usually based, as I mentioned, on what is called parallel play. In this situation two or more children play in close proximity with similar toys or objects but without interacting. At a fundamental level this is not radically different from adult friends who engage in shared activities without interacting. Many times the shared activities of adult friends involve discussions and other interactions, but many times they do not. Or perhaps they involve only minimal interactions. Consider, for example, the adult shared activities of running, trekking, or bicycling (all of which both men and women engage in). Although these may involve conversation or other interaction between the friends, many times they do not. Often the friends simply run or trek in close proximity or, in the case of bicycling, play in close proximity with similar toys (bicycles). The similarity of both the child and adult situation here suggests that the basic human motive behind the friendships might not be too distinct.

Why, then, do small children seek out friendships at all? That is, why do they seek out parallel play situations? Why do they not simply play alone? The basic answer here would seem to be similar to the answer given to the question of why adults seek out friendships at all: namely, that, like adults, children seek out friends to lessen their sense of isolation. This is why they seek out peers rather than just remain with their parents; they are similar to their peers and thus feel less isolated when they are among them. Of course, with the small child the idea of metaphysical isolation will not be fully apparent, but the awareness of simple isolation from others is nevertheless not fully distinct from the awareness of metaphysical isolation.

Returning to the idea of the sense of accessing another person's consciousness, it is natural to think that this is also something that happens in romantic love, marriage, or other close relationships. My feeling, however, is that this is only true so far as such relationships are also instances of friendship. If one's romantic partner or spouse is also one's friend, then all of what has just been said will also be true of one's romantic or marital partner. However, it will only be true by virtue of his or her being one's friend, not because he or she is one's lover, husband, or wife. Many people who are in love are also clearly good friends, even best friends. But, as I have argued, someone can easily be in love with another person without liking that person and therefore without being that person's friend. This seems even more so for marriage, something that can easily lack both love and friendship.

Someone might be tempted to reply that friendship is a natural part of the development of romantic love and marriage, at least if the marriage is going to persist. This is something I will deal with in more depth in Chapter Five. For now, however, I will only point out that such a development need not occur, even if a marriage is to persist. This is obvious from the fact that in many traditional cultures marriages are still arranged by the families of the bride and groom. In some cases, in what are called "blind marriages," the bride and groom never even see each other before the wedding. Here friendship or even love might be wholly absent as a basis for the marriage. Friendship, love, or both might eventually appear as husband and wife get to know each other, but in other cases they might not appear.

Unfortunately, there is little research on the development of friendship in arranged marriages. There are data on marital satisfaction in arranged marriages, which might be indicative of friendship. If it is, then it seems that friendship can develop in such marriages. For people in arranged marriages can report marital satisfaction. For example, in a study comparing marital satisfaction in arranged marriages in India with free-choice marriages in both India and the United States, it was found that those in the arranged marriages in India reported higher marital satisfaction (at least according to a particular questionnaire) than did the free-choice marriages.[26] However, in China, where both free-choice and arranged marriages take place, a study showed that women in free-choice marriages were consistently more satisfied with their marriages, at all points in the marriage, than women in arranged marriages.[27] But again, it is unclear how this should be interpreted in terms of the role of friendship in marriages.

Secondly, even in Western culture, where people can always freely choose their marital partner, some people still see marriage and friendship as being distinct relationships. This view is succinctly stated by a subject in a study by Robert Bell who says, "I don't think that friendship has anything to do with marriage. I wouldn't want my wife to be my best friend. I think as a wife she should respect me and treat me the way a good wife should. For my friends I want other men who can share activities with me and opinions that a woman can't."[28] And it is not just men who can hold such a view. A woman from the same study says, "I have four close women friends. I can be completely honest and self-revealing because they know everything about me. I can talk about all kinds of personal things. I think friendships are more important than marriage. To have no friends would be worse than to have no marriage."[29]

In both these cases what seems to be stopping the person from having a friendship with his or her spouse is the spouse's sex. Thus, the man has the idea that women, and consequently his wife, are incapable of engaging in the sort of sharing that he wants in a friend. Similarly, the woman refers to revelations that she is able to make with her same-sex friends, something that she feels cannot take place in marriage, that is, with a man. In the case of the woman, however, she does not explicitly state that it is the sex of a male marital partner that is the problem. It might, for example, be the marital relationship. Perhaps she could be completely honest and self-revealing to a man who was not her husband. The fact, however, that her close friends are all females does suggest that, for her, it is the sex of her marital partner that would stop her from becoming his friend.

The idea of a cross-sex friend, however, normally refers to men and women who are friends but are not in a romantic, marital, or even sexual relationship. Not surprisingly, here, too, there are people who feel that friendships with the opposite sex are somehow lacking in what they want out of friendship. Or they might even feel that, because of the sex difference or other features that come with the sex differences, such friendships are not really possible. Nevertheless, as stated at the opening of this chapter, the incidence of cross-sex friendships have dramatically increased in recent times. This shows, as does the research in this area, that cross-sex friendships are clearly possible. Further, after listening to what people say about their cross-sex friendships, it is evident that for many people, cross-sex friendships offer a dimension in friendship that is difficult to find in same-sex friendships. What, then, is the nature of cross-sex friendship?

CROSS-SEX FRIENDSHIP

Compared with same-sex friendships, cross-sex friendships have received little scholarly attention. This neglect is peculiar because the idea of a cross-sex friendship is inherently fascinating. What is fascinating about it is simply that it is a warm relationship of mutual liking between a man and a woman that nevertheless does not involve a sexual relationship. Of course, a friendship between a man and woman can involve a sexual relationship. In such a situation the cross-sex friendship has altered in an important way. The friends then become sexual friends. This is something I will explore in the following chapter. For now I will merely say that sexual attraction takes place differently in these two sorts of relationships.

I just said that what is fascinating about the cross-sex friendship is that it nevertheless does not involve a sexual relationship. The reason I say "nevertheless" is because when most people think of a warm relationship of mutual liking between a man and a woman, it seems that what immediately comes to mind is a sexual or romantic relationship. This does not mean that one thinks of such a friendship as necessarily involving an actual sexual relationship, but only that the idea of a man and a woman in a friendship awakens ideas about the man and woman having sex. Perhaps one wonders if they have had sex, if they want to have sex, if they are on their way to a romantic and thus also sexual relationship, and so on. For in most people's minds there seems to be a natural connection between a man and woman's mutual liking in friendship and their having a sexual relationship. At least one can say that the idea of a sexual relationship seems more naturally to come to mind in considering a cross-sex friendship than in considering a same-sex friendship, or at least in a same-sex heterosexual friendship. For if one imagines a same-sex friendship in which both friends are homosexual, then the idea of a sexual relationship might also come to mind. This is because for homosexual persons it is others of the same sex who are typically objects of sexual attraction. This would appear to mean that a same-sex friendship between homosexuals would be somewhat equivalent to a cross-sex friendship between heterosexuals; for both would be friendships in which there seems to be a natural connection between the partner's mutual liking in friendship and a sexual relationship.

However, the little work that has been done on the relation between homosexual same-sex friendships and heterosexual cross-sex friendships does suggest they operate in basically different ways. First, sexual attraction does not typically seem to be present in homosexual same-sex friendships. Secondly, although heterosexual cross-sex friendships often are the soil out of which romantic relationships can grow, the same does not seem to be the case for homosexual same-sex friendships.[30] In addition to this, a recent study suggests other important differences.[31] One is that while heterosexual men often seek out female friends for emotional support, homosexual men do not typically do the same with their male friends. If a homosexual man wants emotional support or to share personal feelings with a friend, he will, like the heterosexual male, tend to choose a female friend. This means that while a heterosexual male will seek emotional support from the sort of friend to whom he could be sexually attracted, a homosexual male will seek emotional support from the sort of friend to whom he is *not* sexually attracted. In other words, if a man wants emotional support, then, whether he is heterosexual or homosexual, he will tend to prefer such support from a female friend. Or, to put it another way, neither heterosexual nor homosexual men turn to male friends for their emotional needs. This suggests that, for heterosexual men, cross-sex friendships are serving needs different from those that same-sex friendships are serving for homosexual men.

Now, although men often see women friends as providers of emotional support, this is only one motive in male attraction to a cross-sex friend. Many men report, for example, that there is a competitiveness in their friendships with other men that is absent in their friendships with women. As a result, a cross-sex friendship can provide a man with a sort of sanctuary in which he can enjoy a friendship without its being tainted by competitive concerns.

Further, as several men have told me, one of the benefits of having close women friends is that, because of the closeness of the friendship, they are able to get a glimpse of the world, as it were, through female eyes. When interacting with his woman friend, a man is able to see how women tend to look at relationships (including friendship), men and women, family, life goals, values, and any other concerns. The psychologist Carol Gilligan, for example, has argued that women typically have a different way of experiencing and construing moral issues than men do.[32] For the man who has a woman friend, he is brought as close as possible to having this female experience.

A man, of course, might easily understand by description a female way of seeing various issues without having a female friend. He can discuss them with women colleagues and other women who are not his friends, read accounts, and so forth. But in having a woman friend, he gets to know this experience by a sort of warm acquaintance, that is, through an intimate interaction in the context of mutual liking, rather than by mere description. This acquaintance is not a direct connection with his cross-sex friend's consciousness. For as I argued earlier, we never have that sort of access to another person's consciousness. But as I also argued, friendship enables us to have the experience of coming as close as possible to such access, something that lessens our sense of metaphysical isolation. This is also true for cross-sex friendship.

However, cross-sex friendships are distinguished from same-sex friendships in a fundamental way, namely, by the existence of sexual attraction. As several studies have shown, it is an element that is present in diverse ways in cross-sex friendships.[33] Various quantitative studies have reported different percentages of cross-sex friends who claim to be sexually attracted to each other (58 percent, 62 percent, and so on). I am, however, doubtful about the accuracy of such statistics, which are often obtained in questionnaires rather than in qualitative interviews or, what is better, direct observation of the couple's interactions (which frequently reveal subtle or even not so subtle signs of sexual attraction). This is because people in cross-sex friendships typically do not want to admit to themselves the sexual attraction they feel for their cross-sex friend. Acknowledging the sexual attraction could be worrying for several reasons. They might feel, for example, that in admitting the sexual attraction, they bring themselves closer to acting on it, which in turn might bring them closer to falling in love. Or maybe they feel it would push the friendship into a phase of uncertainty. And maybe, again for various reasons, they do not want the friendship to develop these ways.

Moreover, as the sociologist J. Donald O'Meara has argued, cross-sex friendships are commonly seen by those outside the friendships as deviant or even threatening.[34] This is because they threaten the traditional view that a man and a woman who like each other and spend time together must really be in a romantic relationship or at least be on the way to it. It is this traditional view that often seems to be the source of problems if either of the cross-sex friends has a romantic or marital partner. For in such a case the romantic partner or spouse might become jealous. He or she might feel the friendship is or could develop into a romance and so threaten his or her own romantic relationship. Or the individual may not like his or her lover seeing another opposite-sexed person because it will look to other people like a sexual affair. It is important to note, however, that having a cross-sex friend while having an understanding and supportive romantic partner—one who is not threatened or jealous—is not unheard of. In such cases it seems the cross-sex friends typically monitor and respond to their romantic partner's reactions to the friendship and attempt to find creative ways to incorporate the friendship into their lives. The research shows, however, that cross-sex friendships are considerably less likely among married and romantically attached persons.[35]

As a result, cross-sex friends face a public relations challenge when they feel pressure to present themselves as friends in an authentic friendship. A convenient way of dealing with all these problems would be simply to deny to others—and why not to oneself while one is at it?—that one has any sexual attraction for one's cross-sex friend. This would seem especially to be the case for females. Females who express such attraction could easily expose themselves to social criticism for being "loose," "an easy lay," or some such undesirable thing. For why does a woman continue to see a man to whom she is sexually attracted if not for the reason of eventually having sex with him? Continuing to see him suggests she has sexual intentions toward someone with whom she has no romantic intentions, which is something women are still criticized for. Consequently, it is no wonder that many surveys have women reporting that they experience less sexual attraction in their cross-sex friendships than men experience, for there is strong social pressure for a woman to deny such attraction, even to herself.

One study found that although the women reported less sexual attraction to their male friends, they nevertheless were quite aware of their male friend's sexual attraction toward them.[36] But the fact that a woman continues in a warm and intimate friendship with a man who she knows is sexually attracted to her suggests that she, too, at some level of awareness, is sexually attracted to him. In some cases it might well be that the woman has no sexual attraction toward the man but merely enjoys his displays of sexual attraction to her. Perhaps his attentions confirm her picture of herself as a sexually attractive woman. But I then would wonder if she would continue to seek out and enjoy this man's warm and intimate company if she found him sexually unattractive or, say, even repulsive. It is nice to have a man find you sexually attractive, but mainly if you yourself find him at least somewhat sexually attractive.

It is not just females, however, who might deny the sexual attraction they feel for their cross-sex friend. For males, too, face social pressure to convince others, and also themselves, that their cross-sex friendship is not just a façade for a sexual liaison. This would particularly be the case if the man also has a romantic partner. In any event, however, the method of choice would seem to be simply to deny that there is any sexual attraction. Although this sort of denial can easily be done on a questionnaire by simply ticking the correct box, this is more difficult to do when being observed, in an interview, or when giving a descriptive account. For in each case denials of sexual attraction often reveal it anyway. Consider the following account from a study on how people construct myths to manage their cross-sex friendships. In this account the man says of his cross-sex friendship:

> I always get a kiss hello and a kiss good-bye—sometimes even more than one. I get kisses sometimes when I do a good thing or sometimes for no reason. In the middle of a conversation, one of us can just walk up to the other and put our arm around the other for no particular reason. When we are by ourselves watching a movie, now and then she will lie against me or I will rest my head on her leg. We will not get the wrong idea, and because we have been friends for such a long time, this abundance of affection just comes natural.[37]

Although it is not fully clear what "get the wrong idea" means, when it is used in discussing something apparently sexual it typically refers to thinking that something is sexual when it is not. That is, to get the wrong idea about a particular behavior is to think the behavior is sexual when in fact it is not. This seems to be the sense in which the man is using it here.

Therefore, even though he and his friend are involved in lots of kissing, hugging, lying against each other, or resting his head on her leg, they do not get the wrong idea. That is, even though they are involved in what are apparently expressions of sexual attraction, they themselves do not get the wrong idea and think that they are sexually attracted to each other.

Now, were this person to answer a question on a survey about whether he was sexually attracted to his cross-sex friend, he would more than likely answer "No" (only if he had the "wrong idea" would he answer "Yes"). Yet from his description it seems fairly evident that there is sexual attraction in this friendship. Further, one can imagine that were he with a man friend, he would probably not get so many kisses, especially for "no reason," or put his arms around him "for no particular reason." Nor would his man friend probably lie against him or he put his head on his man friend's thigh while watching a movie alone with him. Why not? Because in Western culture such actions are typical expressions of sexual attraction and, assuming he is heterosexual, he would not be sexually attracted to his man friend.

Therefore, although he says there is no reason for the extra kisses he gets from his friend or for times when they put their arms around the other, the more plausible explanation is that there is indeed a reason. And this reason is none other than their sexual attraction to each other. In other words, his attempt to explain the "abundance of affection" simply in terms of having been friends for such a long time seems unconvincing. If this was the explanation, then such an abundance should also "come natural" to two men who had been friends for a long time.

The element of sexual attraction might be one of the reasons that cross-sex friendships tend to be more common among young and unmarried people or those not in a romantic relationship.[38] For many people feel their romantic and sexual attachments can only be aimed at one person. These feelings, however, might well be challenged by the sexual attraction that inevitably takes place in a cross-sex friendship. Further, even if the person did not feel this, his or her partner could easily be jealous or unaccepting of the partner's cross-sex friend. A solution to these problems would be to avoid having cross-sex friends.

The element of sexual attraction also means that, for the heterosexual at least, one is at the same time coming as close as possible to the awareness of a person to whom one is sexually attracted. Further, although some men see this attraction as being a burden in the relationship, it is clear that most men value the experience of sexual attraction to and from their cross-sex friend.[39] Before I come to the question of what it means for the friendship to come as close as possible to the awareness of a person to whom one is sexually attracted, let me first turn to the female experience of cross-sex friendships.

First, it should be noted that although women do not follow the male pattern of turning to cross-sex friends for emotional support, they do follow the pattern of turning to *female* friends for such support. And this is true of both homosexual and heterosexual women. Consequently, a woman's sexual orientation does not affect her choice in deciding whether to turn to a male or female friend when she is in need of emotional support or an intimate discussion: in each case she will tend to prefer a female friend. Further, unlike homosexual men or heterosexual women, with lesbians there seems little desire to seek out cross-sex friends. And this is understandable since, being lesbian, they are neither sexually attracted to men nor, like everyone else, do they find men friends to be particularly valuable as providers of emotional support. Also, being themselves women—women who are not sexually attracted to men—if the man is heterosexual, they may well find any sexual interest he might show to be unwelcome.

But if women do not normally seek emotional support from their male friends, what is it they tend to want out of the friendship? Here it is noteworthy that, just like men, women tend to find that their friendships with men are lacking in the competition and jealousy often found in their same-sex friendships.[40] As one of my female students told me, "We are just as competitive as men, but what we compete about is our looks." Therefore, a friendship with a man can offer a woman a place where she can experience mutual liking and companionship without the unpleasantness of rivalries. Similarly, again just like men, many women feel that having a cross-sex friendship enables them to see the world from the opposite-sex's perspective. Interestingly, what many women find bothersome about men as friends, what they variously refer to as men's cognitive or intellectual style, is sometimes what fascinates them about their male friends. This can also, on occasion, be found useful. As one woman says about the male way of dealing with problems, "I have a love-hate relationship to that one-two-three problem-solving mode of theirs. There are times when I can't stand it, and then there are other times when it's exactly what I'm looking for."[41]

Likewise, just as a man can understand a female perspective without having a female friend, so, too, can a woman understand a male perspective without having a male friend. But here, too, she will tend to lack the warm acquaintance with this perspective that has a better chance of being acquired in the intimate relation of a cross-sex friendship. One women I interviewed, a divorced Danish nurse who had no close male friends (though she did have a boyfriend), felt that the lack of such friends made it difficult for her to appreciate a male, and particularly her husband's perspective. She first told me that she had often thought about having a male friend but, for various reasons, never had the chance. When I asked her why she should like to have a male friend, she replied that she thought having such a friend would be helpful in gaining an understanding about men. This understanding was of interest to her because she thought it would have enabled her to get a deeper understanding of her husband. When one is married, she told me, it is difficult sometimes to understand one's partner because there are so many feelings going on. Thus, when she could not understand why her husband did something, she wished she had a man friend she could talk with to help her get some insight into her husband's actions. If she had had such a confidant, she might not have got divorced (or maybe she might have got divorced earlier).

It is noteworthy that this same view, that a male friend might be able to help a woman to understand things about her husband or male partner, is not simply a Western view. This is suggested by a Ugandan woman who, referring to misunderstandings with her husband, said, "My male friends usually tell me what to do whenever I've had misunderstandings; they help me get the male perspective."[42]

It is also clear that, just like men, women tend to value the sexual attraction that takes place in a cross-sex friendship. For many women, the sexual attraction that their man friend shows toward them is seen to validate their self-image as being feminine and sexually attractive to the opposite sex.[43]

We can now come back to a decisive feature of cross-sex friendships that was mentioned earlier. This is the fact that such friendships enable the individual to come close to the awareness of a person of the sexually attractive gender. Since sexual attraction is, as I have argued, fundamentally entangled with the relationship one has to the sexually attractive person, then any sexual attraction that appears will be affected by the cross-sex friendship in which it takes place. Of course, sexual attraction can appear toward a stranger and, as I also tried to show, one's relationship to a stranger will likewise affect any sexual attraction that one might have toward the stranger. A major difference, however, is that in the case of a stranger, one lacks the intimate warmth of mutual liking that one has with a cross-sex friend.

This does not mean that cross-sex friends will necessarily act on the sexual attraction and therefore try to have sex with each other. It seems likely, however, that cross-sex friends who are sexually attracted to each other will have a higher chance of engaging in sex than will strangers or even acquaintances who are similarly attracted. One study discovered that 51 percent of the subjects had engaged in sexual intercourse at least once with a cross-sex friend, while one-third of the subjects had engaged in sexual intercourse repeatedly with such a friend.[44] Although 51 percent or so of people might have similarly engaged at least once with an acquaintance or stranger, it does seem unlikely that one-third of people have engaged in sex repeatedly with the same acquaintance or stranger.

All of this raises several intriguing questions about the relation between cross-sex friendship and sexual attraction. For one, it raises the question of the prevalence of sexual attraction in cross-sex friendships. Because of the number of people eventually having sex with their cross-sex friends, especially repeatedly, it would seem that sexual attraction in cross-sex friendships is fairly prevalent. But, as we have seen, one need not have sexual attraction to another person in order to have sex with him or her. Still, it does not seem unreasonable to suppose that much of the sexual interaction between cross-sex friends has its basis in sexual attraction.

This is further supported by the fact that cross-sex friends—even those not having sex—in many ways match the profile of romantic and thus sexual partners. For example, in cross-sex friendships the man tends to be older and more educated and have a higher-status occupation than the woman.[45] This is also true of romantic partners. Although there are no data here, because of this it would seem likely that cross-sex friends also follow the cardinal principal of dating, that is, that the man must be taller or at least as tall as the woman. In addition, studies show that cross-sex friendships involve significantly more touching than do same-sex friendships,[46] typically flirtatious touching and even explicitly sexual touching.[47] (Here is where cross-sex friendships can move over the blurry border into sexual friendships.)

It is also significant to note that the patterns of touching in cross-sex friendships tend to mirror the patterns of touching in sexual relationships and relationships that are progressing toward becoming romantic relationships. For example, a man tends to find the touch of his woman friend to be sexually arousing, regardless of how intimate the friendship is. However, whether or not a woman finds the touch of her man friend[48] to be sexually arousing will depend on how intimate she finds the friendship to be. In other words, as the intimacy in a cross-sex friendship increases, so does the woman's sexual arousal when touching or being touched by her man friend. Since all of these features tend to be present in sexual and romantic relationships, and since sexual and romantic relationships tend to be infused with sexual attraction, it looks like sexual attraction also plays a fairly basic role in cross-sex friendships.

It would definitely be worthwhile to know if cross-sex friends tended to resemble each other's opposite-sex parent or even resembled each other (which I argued earlier might be a roundabout way of resembling each other's opposite-sex parent). This tends to be the case in romantic and marital partners, who are frequently sexually attracted to one another. Therefore, if cross-sex friends similarly resembled each other's opposite-sex parent, this would be further evidence of the important role of sexual attraction in the friendship. Unfortunately, there seem to be no studies that explore this issue. My feeling, however, is that there would be a tendency for cross-sex friends to show this sort of resemblance.

If this were the case, it would imply that cross-sex friends were chosen, just as sexual partners tend to be chosen, for their sexual attractiveness. Here, though, I would suspect that the role of sexual attractiveness would not be as strong as it would be between romantic partners. The reason I think this is simply that the sexual attraction that takes place among romantic partners plays a more exclusive role in their relationship than does the sexual attraction that takes place among cross-sex friends. This is because in addition to any sexual attraction that cross-sex friends might have for each other, they also have their friendship, which is not necessarily true of romantic partners. Romantic partners, of course, have their romantic love, which cross-sex friends do not, but romantic love is not distinct from a sexual relationship in the way that friendship is. As a result, the sexual attraction that exists between cross-sex friends does not play as decisive a role in the friendship as the sexual attraction that exists between lovers plays in their romance. Even so, my guess would be that a cross-sex friendship that lacked all sexual attraction would be a rare occurrence.

One issue that needs to be addressed with sexual attraction in cross-sex friendships is that of apparent gender differences. Various findings seem to imply that men and women in cross-sex friendships might undergo sexual attraction to each other differently. There are, for example, the just mentioned findings concerning gender differences in touch and sexual arousal in cross-sex friendships. This might be seen to imply that while men are usually sexually attracted to their cross-sex friends, women only become sexually attracted when intimacy in the friendship increases. The problem, however, is that the findings in this study were concerning sexual arousal, not sexual attraction. And one does not have to be sexually aroused in order to experience sexual attraction. This is because the idea of sexual arousal entails the idea of physiological arousal but sexual attraction does not. The experience of sexual attraction might lead to physiological arousal, but there is no reason why it need do so. For one can easily notice the subtle pull of allure while remaining physiologically unaroused. The obvious evidence for this is that one can easily feel the allure of one's sexual partner even after one has had sexual intercourse with him or her and thus is no longer physiologically aroused.

Some studies, however, report that sexual attraction between cross-sex friends is more frequent for the male friend than for the female friend.[49] This might in turn suggest that sexual attraction plays a more important role in cross-sex friendships for men than it does for women. I think, however, that various things likewise count against this suggestion. For example, evolutionary psychologist April Beske-Rechek and her co-workers, the authors of one such study, suggest that perhaps young women are less inclined than men to admit being sexually attracted to a cross-sex friend.[50] Although they try to dismiss this suggestion, I feel it makes sense both in light of the common belief that cross-sex friendships are somehow really sexual relationships and in light of the stigma attached to the idea of a woman who might have sexual relationships with her friends. This seems especially so for a woman who is in a romantic relationship with one man while in a cross-sex friendship with another. Many people, not least her romantic partner, would probably be apprehensive about the cross-sex friendship.

In this regard it seems significant to note that young women who are in a romantic relationship report less sexual attraction toward their cross-sex friends than do women who are not in a romantic relationship (men in a romantic relationship do not report less sexual attraction). This is noteworthy because, in terms of avoiding stigma, it is the type of report that would be expected. For if there is a stigma surrounding the idea of a woman who might have sex with her friends, there would seem to be double the stigma concerning the idea of a woman who might have sex with a friend when she herself is already in a romantic relationship with another man. Such a woman might be seen as "cheating on her man," "two-timing," "untrue," or some such thing. In this case, one way to avoid or at least lessen the stigma would be for the woman to make light of or deny, even to herself, that she had sexual attraction to her cross-sex friend.

It is also suggestive that, in this same study, women reported feeling less sexual attraction to their cross-friends who were in romantic relationships than to those who were not (again, men do not do this). For the question one wants to ask here is, if sexual attraction is based on physical appearance, why should a man be less sexually attractive to his cross-sex friend simply because he is in another relationship? It seems to me that there are at least three likely answers here, and in none of these is it true that the man really becomes less sexually attractive to the woman.

In the first case, the woman is aware of the stigma attached to a woman who maintains a close friendship with a man who is himself romantically involved with another woman. Such a woman could be seen as "trying to steal another woman's man," a "home wrecker," and so forth. Also, the evidence is quite clear that many women in romantic relationships (at least in supposedly nonpolygamous Western culture) do not like their partner seeing another woman, even if the partner and the woman are just friends. It seems likely that the woman friend of a romantically involved man might be uncomfortable with the idea that the man's romantic partner resented his cross-sex friendship. One way for a woman in a cross-sex friendship to deal with these problems is, short of ending the friendship, to insist even to herself that she has little or no sexual attraction toward the romantically attached man friend.

In the second case, which could also be blended with the first, the woman is aware that since her man friend is romantically involved with another woman, he is somehow hindered in becoming sexually involved with her. This makes him not less sexually attractive but simply less available for a possible sexual or romantic relationship with her. He is therefore less "attractive" as possible future partner. These two distinct ideas of attractiveness are easy to confuse, and it is not difficult to understand how a woman in this situation might mistakenly think her sexual attraction to her friend is less than it would be if he was not attached. What is less, however, is merely her attraction to him as a possible sexual or romantic partner.

In a further situation, which could also be blended with either or both of the previous cases, the woman might feel herself to be less sexually attractive to her man friend simply because his romantic attentions are directed toward another woman. "For why," her thoughts might go, "does he continue to be romantically involved with her when he also has an intimacy with me? Might it be that I am less sexually attractive than his romantic partner?" Of course, there could be numerous reasons why the man does not leave his partner to romantically pursue his cross-sex friend, reasons that might have nothing to do with his friend's sexual attractiveness. Nevertheless, in this sort of triangular situation, the woman-friend's comparison of her own sexual attractiveness with that of her man-friend's lover seems a likely occurrence.

In each of these situations I think it is also important to see that none of the foregoing considerations need be clearly laid out in the woman's mind. For example, she need not be openly considering the idea that if her man friend did not have his romantic partner, then she could make a move to embark on a sexual or romantic relationship with him. This might only be a vague or even unconscious consideration that she may never act upon. The same is true for the possible comparison of her own attractiveness with that of the man's partner.

Because of this, I do not feel we are forced to the conclusion that women have less sexual attraction for their cross-sex friends than men do. Further, my discussions with several women on this point indicate that the element of sexual attraction toward a cross-sex friend is fairly prevalent for women.

It thus seems that, for both men and women, sexual attraction is alive and well in cross-sex friendships. This does not mean that sexual attraction will necessarily be present in every cross-sex friendship, but only that there will be a strong tendency for this to be so. And here it seems important to remember two things. First, finding sexual attraction a burden or trying to ignore it in a cross-sex friendship of course does not show it to be absent, rather it shows it to be present. Secondly, it must be recalled that sexual attraction comes in many degrees, from overpowering to barely noticeable. Consequently, people who feel that there is no sexual attraction in their cross-sex friendship, either to or from their cross-sex friend, might well, upon looking more closely, notice a subtle attraction that makes fleeting appearances in various instances. Then again, they might not. It is worth, however, keeping this possibility in mind. For plainly some people can be overtly quick in dismissing or overlooking their sexual experiences. And this is understandable since the awareness of certain sexual feelings can be unpleasant or embarrassing for various people, especially in a culture like ours that has a long and established tradition of seeing sexuality in a negative light. Because of this, sexual attraction, particularly an attraction that someone might find immoral or repulsive, can also take place at an unconscious level. Here the offending attraction is pushed out of awareness and covered up with other feelings and ideas. This is done by someone in order to defend herself from confronting an attraction that she might, for various reasons, find deeply disturbing.

But if it is true that sexual attraction in these friendships is so widespread, what does this say about the perennial question asked of cross-sex friendships, namely, "Can men and women be just friends?"—a question that is meant to ask about the role of sex in a man and woman's friendship. The problem with answering this question is that it is in fact ambiguous and can be interpreted in various ways. Therefore, if one wants to give a meaningful answer, one first has to be clear about which interpretation of the question one is answering.

For example, in one way the question could be a shortened version of the question "Can men and women be friends without also simultaneously having sexual interactions with each other?" Or in another way it could be asking, "Can men and women be friends without one, the other, or both trying or at least intending to turn the friendship into a sexual relationship?" Yet a further interpretation could be that the question is short for "Can men and women be friends without one, the other, or both being sexually attracted each other?" These are but a few of the possible interpretations of the original question. They seem, however, to be the most likely interpretations of "Can men and women ever be just friends?" Or, if there are other likely interpretations, they will probably be very close to one of these.

Turning then to the first interpretation, namely, "Can men and women be friends without also simultaneously having sexual interactions with each other?" the answer seems obvious. For plainly not every cross-sex friendship involves present or even past sexual interactions. Further, as just shown, the available research also supports this view.

What then about the second interpretation? This form of the question also seems easily answered. For although one cannot always be certain about other people's intentions, everyday observation suggests that men and women friends do not always have such intentions. Further, the research indicates that many in these relationships are, on the contrary, concerned that the friendship might develop into a sexual relationship or at least lead the friends into having sex, and so do what they can to avoid such a development. Typically, this is because they believe having sex with their friend would spoil the friendship, change it into an unwanted romance, or at least alter it in an undesirable way. They might also already be in a sexual or romantic relationship with another person and, for whatever reason, not want to embark on another and simultaneous sexual relationship.[51]

There is, however, a slight difficulty in trying to give a definite answer to this second interpretation, that is, to the question "Can men and women be friends without one, the other, or both trying or at least intending to turn the friendship into a sexual relationship?" For just as one cannot always know what someone else's intentions are, so can one not always know what one's own intentions are, or at least be immediately clear what one's own intentions are. This seems to be especially the case where one has feelings of guilt or anxiety over one's intentions. Because of the unpleasantness of such feelings, there is sometimes a tendency to repress and thus conceal them to varying degrees from oneself. This mechanism of hiding one's intentions from oneself can take place in a cross-sex friendship. For here, too, an individual can feel guilty or bothered over his or her sexual desires or intentions toward his or her friend. Perhaps the individual feels that such intentions imply that he or she wants to exploit the friendship or perhaps, as just stated, the individual is already in an exclusive sexual relationship. Thus, he or she might try to sweep the intentions out of awareness or at least try to overlook them. Consequently, when a person reports that she has no sexual intentions toward her cross-sex friend, even though she might be sincere, it cannot be immediately ruled out that she has no such unconsciously hidden intentions.

Still, although it is no doubt true that some people have unconscious intentions to have sex with their cross-sex friends, it seems unlikely that this is always or even mostly true. This is because to intend something, even to intend it unconsciously, is to be committed in some way to carrying it out.[52] However, my discussions with people about their cross-sex friendships along with other research suggests that many such people have no form of commitment to having sex with their cross-sex friend. If someone had an unconscious commitment to having sex with her cross-sex friend, it seems that this commitment would eventually affect her behavior (for this is how we know about unconscious intentions—and their commitments), and there would be some form of display of such a commitment. But I have seen no evidence that this is always or even mostly the case.

This brings us to the third interpretation of the question, namely, "Can men and women be friends without one, the other, or both being sexually attracted each other?" Of the three interpretations of the question, this one stands out as being the best candidate for receiving a negative answer. This is because, as I have argued throughout this study, sexual attraction is widespread. Before I try to give a full answer to this question, it will help to examine the typical sort of reasons given by those who might give the answer "No."

A good place to start is with a popular film where the protagonist attempts to answer the question "Can men and women be just friends?" while interpreting the question in more or less the same way as my third interpretation. The film I have in mind is *When Harry Met Sally*, a film well known for the claim made by the male protagonist that men and women cannot be friends (by which he seems to mean "just friends"). This happens during a dialogue between the two main characters, Harry and Sally, when Sally, who is concerned over Harry's sexual attraction to her, tells him, "We are just going to be friends, OK?" To this Harry finally replies, "Men and women can't be friends because the sex part always gets in the way." He later tries to qualify this answer, saying, "They can't be friends, unless both of them are involved with other people, then they can. This is an amendment to the earlier rule. The two people are in relationships: the pressure of possible involvement is lifted." He quickly, however, rejects his own qualification, explaining thus:

> That doesn't work either because what happens then is the person you're involved with can't understand why you need to be friends with a person you're just friends with, like it means something is missing from the relationship, and why do you go outside to get it. Then when you say, "No, no, no, no, it's not true, nothing is missing from the relationship," the person you are involved with then accuses you of being secretly attracted to the person you are just friends with, which you probably are, I mean, come on, who the hell are we kidding, let's face it. Which brings us back to the early rule before the amendment, which is men and women can't be friends.

We are thus given two reasons why men and women can't be just friends. The first is that at least one of the persons in the friendship would be secretly attracted to the other. (Harry's earlier comment that "the sex part always gets in the way" make it clear he means "secretly sexually attracted.") The second reason, which only applies when the person is in a romantic relationship with someone else, is that the person's romantic partner will accuse the person of being secretly sexually attracted to his or her friend. The implication of this last reason seems to be that the person's romantic partner will be jealous and not allow the friendship to continue or at least make it difficult. In either case, however, the basic reason why men and women cannot be just friends is that there will always be sexual attraction.

On the point about the presence of sexual attraction in cross-sex friendships, the protagonist seems to be correct. For as I have argued, sexual attraction in these friendships is pervasive. But why should this mean that women and mean cannot be just friends? The unspoken assumption behind this reasoning is clearly that friendship and sexual attraction are somehow incompatible. But is this true? In one obvious sense, friendship and sexual attraction plainly are compatible because many men and women who are in romantic relationships are also often friends, a relationship I will discuss further in Chapter Five. The idea here, however, seems to be that if a man and a woman who are not romantically or sexually involved try to enter into a friendship, sexual attraction will "get in the way" and stop the relationship from being just a friendship.

But why should it get in the way? Unfortunately, the protagonist never tells us why. There seem, however, to be two possible answers here. The first is that sexual attraction could get in the way of the friendship because it leads to the friends' having sex with each other. Once this has happened, it could be argued, then either or both of the friends will no longer see the relationship as primarily a friendship, and begin to view each other as primarily a sexual or romantic partner.

This situation, in which cross-sex friends have sex with each other, is the sexual friendship I referred to earlier. It is something I will examine in the next chapter and so will leave the discussion until then. For now, however, I will merely underscore what I have said at other points in this study, namely, that sexual attraction does not inevitably lead to sexual interaction. There is, as mentioned, a more likely chance that it will lead to sexual interaction in the case of cross-sex friends than in the case of, say, strangers. But still, as the research suggests, although there are a substantial number of cross-sex friendships that involve sexual interaction, there are also a substantial number of cross-sex friendships that do not involve this. It is also quite clear that in many cross-sex friendships the friends are concerned that the attraction will lead to sexual activity, do not want the relationship to turn into a sexual one, and actively take steps to avoid it from happening. If, then, the purported reason why men and women cannot be just friends is that they will end up having sex with each other, then plainly men and women can be just friends. For it is not true that their sexual attraction will inevitably or even usually lead to their having sex.

A second possible view is that, even if sexual attraction does not lead to having sex, it will still spoil the friendship by getting either or both of the friends to see each other as a *potential* sexual or romantic partner. The problem with this answer, however, is it is unclear why seeing someone in this way is incompatible with also being his or her friend. It will be recalled, for example, that in the earlier discussion of the nature of friendship, I pointed to the core elements of friendship as being reciprocity, well-wishing and well-doing for the each other's sake, an awareness of each other's feelings in this regard, and the enjoyment of each other's company or companionship. I do not see that viewing one's friend as a potential sexual partner goes against any of these core elements.

Further, I mentioned that in describing the nature of friendship, people will variously refer to such things as trust, openness, honesty, safety, support, loyalty, constancy, understanding, shared activities, and acceptance. Here, too, there is nothing incompatible with seeing one's friend as a potential sexual partner. I can trust and be open with someone I see as a potential sexual partner, I can be honest with and offer safety, support, and loyalty to someone I see as a potential sexual, and so on. One can easily have all these elements in a friendship with a person one sees as a potential sexual partner.

Of course, one could be secretive and dishonest with one's friend about one's sexual attraction, or one could be secretive and devious in trying to seduce one's friend. In this case, one might well be acting in a way that was incompatible with these elements of friendship. But this is not a problem with sexual attraction or seeing one's cross-sex friend as a potential sexual partner. It is rather a problem about being open and honest. For there is no reason why one cannot be open about one's sexual attraction and about having a sexual view of one's friend. As a result, sexual attraction is quite compatible with friendship and, as I have argued, widely present in cross-sex friendships. This would suggest that the answer to the question "Can men and women be friends without one, the other, or both being sexually attracted each other?" is "Probably not." This, as I said, is the most likely interpretation of the question "Can men and women be just friends?" However, because of the extreme ambiguity of the question, it is safest to avoid giving an answer to such a question until its meaning is clarified.

It is important to keep this interpretation in mind when considering the question of whether men and women can be just friends. This is because it is easy to think the question is asking about whether men and women can be friends at all. The reason is that it is easy to mistakenly think that the expression "just friends" means basically the same as the term "friends." Consequently, someone might think that the question "Can men and women be *just* friends?" is asking the same thing as "Can men and women be friends?" This seems to be the mistake that the protagonist makes in *When Harry Met Sally*. He claims that men and women cannot be friends because "the sex part" (sexual attraction) gets in the way. But as I have shown, friendship and sexual attraction are quite compatible. Consequently, men and women can be friends, it is just that the friendship will more than likely contain sexual attraction. And because friendship and sexual attraction are compatible, there is no reason why "the sex part" need get in the way.

Because of this compatibility of sexual attraction and cross-sex friendships, and because of the ubiquity of sexual attraction in cross-sex friendships, a new way of understanding cross-sex friendships immediately suggests itself. This is the idea that far from being a side effect or unplanned result of cross-sex friendship, sexual attraction might well be a foundational element in the relationship. In this view, sexual attraction is one of the basic elements that initially bring cross-sex friends together. Thus, rather than being an element that haphazardly appears later in the friendship, it could be considered a starting point from which the friendship grows and also an element that continues in various degrees throughout the friendship. This is not to claim that it is the only element in getting the friendship going, for plainly there can be many other features of an opposite-sex person (for example, humor, kindness, trustworthiness) that draw one into a friendship with him or her. It is only to claim that sexual attractiveness is one such basic feature. Such a view is also supported by the fact that sexual attraction plays a foundational role in many sexual interactions, romantic attachments, and many other relationships between men and women. It would therefore be strange if it did not also play such a role in cross-sex friendships.

Even so, it must be noted that sexual attraction can be a starting point in different ways. In one situation someone might find an opposite-sex person sexually attractive and so pursue him or her as a possible sexual or romantic partner. This pursuit, however, for any number of reasons, might not have worked out. Here the interpersonal contact that resulted from the pursuit could have been enough to lead to a cross-sex friendship. In another situation, one or both of the persons may experience sexual attraction but be unsure of whether to proceed to a sexual relationship. Nevertheless, they could still much enjoy each other's company and so, for the time being, continue in a cross-sex friendship. Yet a further situation might be that despite their sexual attraction to each other, neither of the friends wants the friendship to involve a sexual relationship. Again, this could be for many different reasons. In any of these and many other situations, sexual attraction can easily be the starting point of the friendship.

This view, however, goes against that of many scholars. Such people feel that sexual attraction can only be an effect and not a cause of cross-sex friendships.[53] Panayotis Halatsis and Nicolas Christakis, for example, claim that since same-sex friendships provide a model for understanding cross-sex friendships, and since the definition of same-sex friendships presumes the absence of sexual attraction, then the definition of the cross-sex friendships must also presume the absence of sexual attraction. Therefore, they continue, "that sexual attraction cannot be the starting point and foundation of a cross-sex friendship is taken for granted."[54]

But this is an unpersuasive argument. For even if same-sex friendships are used as a model for understanding cross-sex friendships, it is obvious that cross-sex friendships are different in basic ways from same-sex friendships. As a result, one should not expect that all that is true of same-sex friendships (for example, the absence of sexual attraction as a foundational starting point) will be true of cross-sex friendships.

Halatsis and Christakis try to support their argument by asserting, "If the goal of one or both of the members of the dyad is to sexually approach the other sex 'friend,' then the friendly approach is nothing but a kind of 'Trojan horse' for the attainment of erotic purposes."[55] But this assertion also has problems. First, although they start by discussing sexual attraction in this passage, they then switch to the term "sexually approach," as if the two were the same thing. But to have sexual attraction to someone is not the same as to sexually approach him or her. The idea of sexually approaching someone carries with it the idea of trying to get the other person to engage in sex activity, or at least to display one's sexual intentions. Yet the idea of sexual attraction need not involve either of these.

Secondly, it is obvious that, as was discussed earlier, people are multifaceted in what they enjoy and what they require out of a friendship. Consequently, there is no reason why someone need only have one goal in his or her friendship. Therefore, "if the goal of one or both of the members of the dyad is to sexually approach the other sex 'friend,'" this in no way implies that the friendly approach "is nothing but a kind of 'Trojan horse' for the attainment of erotic purposes," for there is no reason why this goal should be their only goal.

It will be recalled that in the earlier discussion of friendship I argued that a basic motivation in friendship is the attempt to overcome a deep-rooted sense of metaphysical isolation. This is also true for cross-sex friendships. However, with cross-sex friendships there is the additional basic motivation of sexual attraction. It seems significant to note, therefore, that the attempt to overcome metaphysical isolation and sexual attraction are not completely unrelated. This becomes evident when it is remembered that the experience of allure involves the image of oneself brought together in physical intimacy with the sexually attractive person. But this idea of being brought together with another person is also what occurs in the attempt to overcome metaphysical isolation through friendship. In friendship, however, the idea refers to being brought together with the thoughts, ideas, and feelings of an individual one deeply understands and whose company one enjoys. Thus, cross-sex friendship has at its core the goal to unify with another person in these two distinct ways. It is this combination that gives the allure of the cross-sex friend its distinct quality.

THE ALLURE OF CROSS-SEX FRIENDS

The fascinating thing about the allure felt toward a cross-sex friend is the way that it is mixed with the attraction of friendship. When I feel allure toward my cross-sex friend, what I am allured by is her sexually attractive physical appearance. In the moment I find her alluring, I feel myself drawn helplessly toward her. The goal of this sensation of being pulled toward her presents itself to my awareness as a sexual fantasy of our two bodies intimately joined. Yet at the same time I am also aware of the attraction of friendship. Consequently, in that same instant I am also aware of our mutual well-wishing and well-doing for each other's own sake, the fun and enjoyment we have in our company and thus companionship, and so on. Of course, I need not at each moment be equally aware of both the allure and the feelings of friendship. I may, for example, be more aware on one occasion of the allure she has for me: perhaps she is wearing something particularly striking or crosses her legs in an alluring way. Or on another occasion I may be more aware of our feelings of friendship than of her allure. Maybe at this moment we are deeply enjoying an intimate and absorbing conversation with each other or perhaps walking together through the fields.

Nevertheless, in each case both types of awareness are present. When it is her allure that is foremost in my awareness, I am still aware, at least in some form, that it is my friend who is casting her allure over me. Thus, in being allured by the crossing of her legs, I am still aware that these are not the legs of just anybody, or of a stranger—of a Mrs. Nobody going nowhere, as the poet says. Nor are they the legs of a romantic partner. Rather, they are the legs of my close friend, someone with whom I experience companionship and thus whose company I enjoy and who enjoys my company. Yet within my experience of the moment, which is dominated by her allure, my awareness of her as my friend retreats into the background. It does this, however, by not simply becoming a weaker form of awareness, but rather by becoming a background awareness that frames and presents her allure in the foreground.

A good way to see what is going on here would be to compare this experience to that of viewing a painting, say a portrait. If we consider, for example, the *Mona Lisa* by Leonardo da Vinci, we will see that the painting is composed of at least two things. These are the image of the woman in the foreground and the background that surrounds her. Now, although the background plays a secondary role in how we initially view the painting, it nevertheless has an important effect. It is the woman, of course, with her penetrating gaze and indiscernible smile, who catches the focus of our attention. But the surrounding background nevertheless works to give a context in which the woman is presented. And even though the viewer of the painting might direct her attention to the image of the woman, the background nevertheless seeps into the viewer's focused awareness, as it were, from the periphery of the painting. The background in the *Mona Lisa* is a peculiar one, namely, a barren and rocky landscape with a winding road and a bridge that seems to go nowhere. There is a lake, but rather than being surrounded by greenery, it looks more like a crater on the moon that has been filled with water. This background creates a surrealistic context that works to give the woman an other-worldly quality, somehow lifting her from the natural world and transforming her into a mythical and thus timeless being.

Now, if this way of understanding a painting is compared with that of understanding the relation between allure and friendship within a cross-sex friendship, some interesting points of similarity emerge. For just as the background of the portrait is separate from the image of the person in the portrait, so is the friendship we feel for a cross-sex friend separate from the allure of the cross-sex friend. And just as the background nonetheless goes on to affect our perception of the person in the portrait, so does the attraction of friendship nonetheless go on to affect the friend's allure. With the *Mona Lisa* the surrealistic background affects our perception of the woman by imparting a sense of surrealism to her. With a cross-sex friendship the warmth and closeness of friendship affects the allure of the cross-sex friend by imparting a sense of warmth and closeness to the allure. How does it do this? In the same way that the awareness of the background in the *Mona Lisa* affects the awareness of the image of the woman, namely, by seeping in from the peripheral feelings of friendship to surround the experience of allure. In doing so, however, it does not alter the structure of allure. Listening to people's accounts of the allure they feel toward a cross-sex friend, I find that the components of feeling drawn, a sense of helplessness, and the fantasies of sexual contact are easily discernible. Yet it also seems clear that these components of the allure are affected by the friendship felt toward the alluring person.

If we examine the component of the sense of being drawn, it is evident that the person I am being drawn to is someone with whom I have close feelings of friendship. What I am being drawn to, within the experience of allure, is her sexually attractive appearance. But since she is already my friend, I am at the same time aware of the mutual liking we have for each other, and that draws me toward her as a friend. This attraction to her as a friend, however, is not sexual attraction to her physical appearance, but rather to the well-wishing and well-doing she bears toward me, to her sense of humor, kindness, companionship, and so forth. These feelings of friendship provide a warm and protective environment through which I can sense myself being drawn toward my friend. It might be compared to being swept along in a current of warm water, where the current is the sense of being drawn and the warm water is the warmth of friendship.

This contrasts starkly with the allure of a stranger about whom I know nothing save her physical appearance. As I mentioned in the last chapter, this creates the effect of enticing one forward in a purely impersonal way. Here, there is no warmth or closeness that surrounds or bathes the sense of being drawn. This gives the magnetic pull of the alluring stranger a pure and undiluted quality. With the cross-sex friend, however, the feeling of being drawn is experienced in the midst of mutual liking and so seems supported by it. This is because the alluring sense of being drawn is not at all adverse to the attraction of liking. On the contrary, it seems to complement it. For both imply a coming together of two people. Of course, the sense of being drawn in allure seems to take place of its own accord, with little interest in whether one likes the alluring individual as a friend. But the fact remains that the sense of being drawn in allure is, as with the attraction of friendship, still a positive movement toward another person. This seems enough to create a link between the two experiences, allowing the feelings of friendship to provide a particular environment for the experience of this component of allure.

It is, however, important to note two things here. First, the fact that one enjoys the attraction of friendship with one's cross-sex friend does not imply that one will enjoy the sense of being sexually drawn to one's cross-sex friend. Research shows that many people find the sexual attraction in their cross-sex friendships to be a burden or to create an uncomfortable tension. I would take this as evidence for the idea that some people react in a negative way to the pull of allure toward their cross-sex friend.

My impression, however, is that most who have this negative experience are in fact feeling ambivalent. That is, although in one sense they experience this pull of allure in a negative way, in another sense they experience it positively. This would be simply because, in itself, the sense of being drawn in allure toward an attractive person of the opposite sex is typically (though not always) a positive experience. As a result, if other considerations give the experience a negative dimension—considerations such as fear that sex would spoil the friendship, change it into an undesired romance, or some such thing—this would not completely remove the positive dimension of the experience but rather create an unpleasant ambivalence.

Secondly, the fact that an opposite-sex person is one's friend will, in itself, tend not to affect the intensity of being alluringly drawn to him or her. This is because, as I have argued previously, allure has its basis in the person's sexually attractive physical appearance. Consequently, what one finds alluring about one's cross-sex friend, and therefore what creates the sense of being sexually drawn to him or her, is his or her physical appearance, not his or her friendship.

This can be at times a difficult distinction to make in the case of a cross-sex friend. The reason for this is simply that both the cross-sex friendship and the elements of allure are in this case experiences of attraction toward the same person. As a result, someone might be tempted to think that the friendship he or she has with an opposite-sex individual somehow increases his or her feelings of sexual attraction to the friend and hence intensifies the sense of being alluringly drawn to the friend. But if this were true, it would seem to imply that the less of a friend someone was, the less one would feel the alluring sense of being drawn to that person. Yet the sense of being sexually drawn to the stranger—to whom one has no friendly feelings—can be just as intense.

There is, however, an area in cross-sex friendship where the distinction between being drawn by friendship and being drawn by physical appearance becomes a bit unclear. This is the area of touching. For as we have seen, cross-sex friendships typically involve a fair amount of touching. But touching can be both a friendly behavior and a sexual behavior. It is friendly when it expresses liking or, say, gives supportive comfort, and it is sexual when it expresses sexual desire or sexual attraction. And, as is well known, it is notoriously difficult to draw an exact line between these two sorts of touching, especially since one instance of touching can easily express both of these motives. Now, since cross-sex friendships involve much touching, touching that could be friendly touching, sexual touching, or touching that was both friendly and sexual, this seems to be an area where part of the friendship could affect the intensity of the allure. In such a case we could imagine that one of the friends touches the other in a way that was meant to be friendly, but which the other friend interprets as sexual. Or the touch could have been both friendly and sexual at the same time. But why should this sort of touch increase the intensity of allure? The reason is that touching is also an observation—a tactile observation—of the other person's physical appearance. That is, when a man, for example, touches his cross-sex friend's hand in a gesture of friendship, he might well suddenly notice the sexual attractiveness of her soft and smooth skin. This might then increase the allure she already has over him.

Turning now to allure's component of helplessness, it is plain that this is also affected by the feelings of friendship. But here, too, as with the sense of being drawn, the feelings of friendship provide a context in which the sense of helplessness takes place. In the case of an alluring stranger, the helplessness has a purity about it, for there is nothing one knows about the stranger other than his or her physical appearance. The sensation of helplessness at being drawn toward the alluring stranger is therefore set in a context where it is uncomplicated by any knowledge one could have about the person; for to be a stranger is to be more or less unknown.

This is in sharp opposition to the context of the helplessness one feels in being sexually drawn toward a cross-sex friend. For in the case of the cross-sex friend, one is indeed in a context that is complicated by other factors, namely, by the feelings of friendship. Consequently, although the allure of one's cross-sex friend creates a sense of helplessness, it is nevertheless before one's kind and caring friend that one feels this helplessness. This does not change the sense of helplessness itself: people can still feel deeply helpless in being allured by their cross-sex friend. It does, however, tend to make the sense of helplessness not as much of a concern. For one need not be so concerned about feeling helplessly drawn to someone who wishes you well and does what she can to bring about your well-being. One could say that the sense of helplessness thus takes place in a safe haven, namely, in the warmth and enjoyment of mutual liking.

It will be recalled that in the earlier discussion of friendship it was mentioned how safety was often seen as an element of friendship. It is in this aspect of cross-sex friendships that we see a natural home for this element. One woman I discussed cross-sex friendships with referred repeatedly to how safe she felt with her cross-sex friend. When I asked her if she could explain what she meant by feeling safe, she replied that although she did feel sexually attracted to him, his kindness to her meant she did not have to worry about those feelings of loss of control. His friendship provided a refuge in which she could have her sexual attraction to him and, whatever happened, even if they had sex, he would still care for her.

The third element of allure is the sexual fantasies that are provoked by the appearance of the sexually attractive person. These are the brief fantasies that involve one's own body being brought intimately together with the other person. This component is also discernible in the allure that people have to their cross-sex friends. As mentioned earlier, with strangers there is the feature of unknownness that affects the fantasy component of allure. For a stranger is typically someone with whom there has been no physical closeness or intimacy. Consequently, one has only a limited exposure to her body, with not much idea concerning the feeling or texture of her skin, the scent of her hair, or the experience of hugging or kissing her. This unknownness naturally affects the sexual fantasies that one forms under her allure. For in lacking this knowledge, the fantasies are limited in the concrete images from memory that they can build upon.

Things, however, are different with the alluring fantasies of a cross-sex friend. Not surprisingly, cross-sex friends spend much more time together than strangers do and, to be sure, in much closer contact. Hugging, flirtatious touching, and sexual touching are common behaviors between cross-sex friends. As a result, there is a wealth of material to fuel sexual fantasies and also to provide images and ideas for the fantasies of allure. It should be noted, however, that although this material will help in the creation of sexual fantasies, the fantasies will nevertheless tend to go beyond such touching and hugging. This is because allure is about sexual attraction, and in such attraction one is drawn to the idea of having sex with the attractive person. The physical interactions of cross-sex friends, however, are not generally seen as instances of having sex (though, as I mentioned, in some cases it might be unclear where to draw the line). And, in being sexually attracted to one's cross-sex friend, one is attracted to an interaction that one can see as having sex. Consequently, the images of touching might become embellished to make them more explicitly sexual. The images taken from earlier interactions, however, will be particularly useful in the embellishment. This is because we know that people tend to fantasize about past or current sexual partners and the specific sexual interactions they have had with them. Although cross-sex friends are not sexual partners, they are nevertheless opposite-sex persons who are sexually attracted to each other and frequently touch each other. Accordingly, the images of their touching can easily be used to provide the raw material that the fantasy can then go on to embellish with more explicit sexual content—perhaps removing the clothes when the hugging and touching takes place or altering a greeting hug into an embrace during sexual intercourse.

But why should people fantasize mainly about past or current sexual partners and the specific sexual interactions they have had with them? A probable answer here is that past, especially recently past, and highly arousing sexual experiences provide readily available images that can be easily woven into a fantasy. They also have the advantage of making the fantasy more connected to reality and thus seem potentially attainable. People do, of course, fantasize about having sex with famous people and other unlikely situations. But these fantasies are far less common. The obvious reasons for this are, first, that the fantasizer has little concrete material upon which to base the fantasy and, secondly, that the fantasy has little chance of ever becoming actual. It is also true, however, that having little concrete material to build upon such fantasies seems to create a wider scope for development. That is, they are less constrained by reality and so able to contain a wider range of exciting images. Although this might seem like a reason for preferring sexual fantasies about strangers, the fact remains that people seem to prefer sexual fantasies with firm ties to reality. And plainly, with a cross-sex friend there is much more reality to tether our fantasies to than with a stranger.

This also seems to hold for the brief fantasies of allure, the fantasies that appear as the goal to which the sense of helplessly being drawn is leading the attracted person.

Thus, when a woman, for example, is suddenly allured by the bare arms of her man friend, she might well recognize the arms as those that she held onto when she reached up to greet him with a kiss, as the arms that rubbed up against her as they went on a walk, and as the arms that firmly hugged her when they last said goodbye. She would therefore have come to know those arms well. These images and sensations of his arms are consequently ready material for use in the fantasy component of allure. Since, however, her past interactions with his arms have not been in an instance of having sex, her fantasy might well take images of her interactions with his arms and enhance these images, making them images of full sexual interaction. Thus, it could easily be that by the allure he emanates toward her, she not only feels herself helplessly drawn toward him, but further has an immediate sexual fantasy of his bare arms picking up her naked body, lifting her into him, holding her in sexual intercourse, or some such thing. It would be these briefly fantasized (and embellished) images that would present themselves to her as the goal to which she feels helplessly drawn.

Further, even though the embellished parts of the images never really happened, because of her intimate knowledge of his arms, the fantasy of his arms holding onto her would still be moderately tethered to reality. This in turn would give such fantasies a degree of realism and of being potentially attainable. For if she has already been hugged by her cross-sex friend, then, her thoughts might go, it is not too unlikely that she might one day be hugged by those arms in a naked embrace. At least it is far more likely than being nakedly embraced by the arms of the alluring stranger she saw at the cinema two days ago.

It is this realism of the sexual fantasies and thus their seeming potential for taking place in reality that gives the allure of a cross-sex friend one of the qualities that distinguishes it from the allure of a stranger. When this is taken together with the fact that the sense of being drawn is felt in a context of warmth and mutual liking, and the sense of helplessness is felt as helplessness before someone kind and caring, then it can be easily understood how the allure of a cross-sex friend takes a firm and yet pleasurable grip on the awareness of the attracted person. It is no great surprise that the borderland between that of a cross-sex friendship without sexual relations and a cross-sex friendship with sexual relations is easily crossed. When this happens, the relationship transforms into a sexual friendship. This will be the subject of the next chapter.

FOUR

More than Just Friends

SEXUAL FRIENDSHIP

When someone has sex with his or her cross-sex friend, the friendship has altered in a basic way. Yet at the same time it seems a completely smooth and natural progression. For as we have seen, sexual attraction is one of the fundamental motivations behind a cross-sex friendship, and indeed cross-sex friendships often take place in a sexual atmosphere of mutual touching, including flirtatious and sexual touching. In this way it seems that cross-sex friendships carry with them subtle, or not so subtle, indications that the friendship might well move toward becoming a new sort of relationship. One thing that could happen is that the friends could fall in love and become romantic partners. However, this is only one possibility. Another is that they could start having sex with each other without falling in love and while still remaining close friends. In another case, after they have started having sex, they might also eventually move on to falling in love. They could even do this while staying friends. But if this happens, then their relationship would also be a romantic one. Further, because of the vital importance that most people attach to falling in love, it seems that the relationship would primarily be seen as a love relationship, albeit one in which the lovers were also friends.

In the case of friends who have sex, but do not fall romantically in love, the friendship might continue and be seen primarily as a friendship, but one in which the friends also have sex. The fact that the friendship is often seen as being primary in such relationships is well expressed in the term that is commonly used to refer to cross-sex friends in these circumstances. This is the term "friends with benefits," where such friends are typically described as being in a "friends with benefits relationship." Here the term "benefits," which is used to describe the sexual part of the relationship, is meant to show that the sex is an extra part of the relationship, rather than the main purpose or core of the relationship.

Although the term "friends with benefits" does have this advantage and is now widely accepted and used in the research that studies these relationships, it is not without its pitfalls. First, it is something of a humorous term that can easily be seen as trivializing or even looking down on the sexual component of the relationship. The implication is that any sex that takes place in cross-sex friendships is merely a perk—like the loan of a car from an employer—rather than anything important itself. But why would anybody want to imply this? Most likely because of the prevailing moralistic view that sex that takes place outside of romantic love is somehow deficient or improper. In these relationships, then, the sex is stigmatized as just being merely a "benefit" rather than being seen as something that enriches or adds to the friendship in an important way. Because of this, it is probably best that scientific research avoid such a term.

A further problem, which is more of a practical one, is that when one wants to refer to the relationship that friends with benefits have, people typically refer to a "friends with benefits relationship." This, however, seems a long and awkward expression, so much so that many researchers have opted for the abbreviated version "FWB relationship." But this is also an awkward term and, in addition, is one whose meaning is not immediately clear to those not involved in the research.

Other terms that have been used—excluding openly derogatory terms—include "flovers,"[1] or "partners in friendship love."[2] But these have the complication of being ambiguous. For again it is not immediately evident if the words within these terms, "lovers" or "love," refer to a sexual or psychological relationship, for the terms "lovers" and "love" in their everyday usage can refer to either love or sex. A lover can be someone with whom one is in love or, more simply, someone with whom one just as sex. Similarly "love" can refer to being in love or to having sex, as in "Do you want to make love?" To avoid these problems, I prefer to use the terms "sexual friends" and "sexual friendship." These expressions strike me as being instantly clear and capturing the basic features of both the members in the relationship and the relationship itself in a neutral and simple way.

Now, just as there are people who find the sexual attraction in a cross-sex friendship disturbing, so are there people who would find sex in a cross-sex friendship disturbing, or even horrifying. For many people the idea of friendship and sex just do not go together. In other words, such people think individuals cannot be both sexual partners and friends with each other, or at least that there is something perverse about doing so. I wonder, though, how much this idea is influenced by thinking of friendship primarily in terms of same-sex heterosexual friendships. For, on the face of it, same-sex heterosexual friendships and having sex do not seem to go together. If someone is thinking of friendship primarily in this way, then it is possible that when he comes to think of a cross-sex friendship, he thinks it ought to be basically the same thing as a same-sex friendship. In such a view, cross-sex friendships are seen to be much like same-sex friendships, with the difference that the friends are opposite sexes (which could then make them seen as deficient approximations to the primary same-sex form of friendship). Nevertheless, since sex has no place in a same-sex friendship, the reasoning would go, then obviously it has no place in a cross-sex friendship, which is, after all, an approximation of a same-sex friendship.

If, however, one discards this way of thinking and sees sexual attraction as a basic motivation in cross-sex friendships—a motivation that is lacking in same-sex friendships—then the idea that friendship and having sex do not go together does not seem so obvious. For plainly, having sex is something that men and women often engage in because of their sexual attraction to each other. Another factor that perhaps stands in the way of accepting the idea of sexual friendship is that this form of relationship has only recently come to most people's attention. Here again, several films and television series from the 1990s onward have slowly brought the idea of sexual friendships into prominence. Thus, films like *Up in the Air*, *No Strings Attached*, and *Friends with Benefits* all portray sexual friendships. Interestingly enough, as with films about cross-sex friendships, the majority of these portraits show the sexual friendship to be impracticable, with one or both of the characters finally falling in love (and attaching strings).

Within the scholarly community, too, a full awareness of the idea of sexual friendships has only appeared in the last decade. Scholarly studies focusing on the topic first started to be published in the early 2000s (though the phenomenon is mentioned before that). A likely explanation for all this is that, again, sexual friendships, like cross-sex friendships, have only recently started appearing, at least in any notable number. In the 1950s, for example, the concept seems more or less nonexistent. And this is understandable, for, as we have seen, cross-sex friendships were themselves nearly nonexistent. And with next to no cross-sex friendships, there can be only be next to no sexual friendships. Therefore, in a sense, the acceptance of cross-sex friendships paved the way for sexual friendships. This does not mean there was no such thing as having sex with friends before the common appearance of cross-sex friendships. For in those uncommon instances of such friendships, which might well have had to be furtive and kept low key, there was probably furtive sex. It is noteworthy to realize, however, that before the recent idea of sexual friendship, people in these relationships would not have had the concept readily available to account for their relationship. Consequently, they would have been under mental pressure to explain their relationship, if only to themselves, as some sort of romantic relationship even though it was clear it was not. This would no doubt have been baffling as they struggled to understand their relationship, which did not easily fit into accepted categories.

Before the common existence of cross-sex friends, the usual partners for sex were seen to be either romantic partners or casual acquaintances or relative strangers (as in the one-night stand). This is not to say that sex in any of these relationships was generally morally approved of. Many people, especially in America, saw and still see marriage (whether or not it involves romantic love) as the only proper place for having sex. It is, however, to say that at least people saw these as the typical relationships in which sex takes place. It might well be the lingering of this conceptual scheme that also plays a part in the widely held idea that friendship and sex do not go together.

It is important to also note here that in many non-Western cultures, sexual friendships could never take place for the simple reason that cross-sex friendships are forbidden. And just as with cross-sex friendships, even in cultures where sexual friendships are neither illegal nor religiously forbidden, there can still be strong social sanctions for anyone who might contemplate such a friendship. In China, for example, there is no legal or religious prohibition against sexual friendships. Yet a 26-year-old male student of mine from Chengsha in central China told me that not only was there no such thing as sexual friendships in China, but the concept did not even exist in China. If a man and woman were to attempt to embark on this type of relationship, no one would accept that it was a friendship. They would see it as simply a dating relationship or at least the preliminary way to one. If the friends were able to convince others that they were not dating or romantically involved, and were simply close friends who also enjoyed having sex, then the social sanctions would start. People would, for example, say they were "crazy," as he put it, and that something was desperately wrong. Furthermore, the girl would be straight away seen as and called a *biao zi* (a derogatory word for a woman who indiscriminately has sex with anyone).

This would especially be so if the woman had more than one sexual friend. In either case, he assured me, her parents would be deeply ashamed and more than likely disown her.

The current situation in Western countries is not this oppressive, and in some social environments, like the university campus, sexual friendships are gaining acceptance. Still, the wider cultural norms are definitely against of this type of relationship. In 1989 O'Meara pointed out that cross-sex friends struggle to have their friendship "while enmeshed in a cultural context that imposes severe limitations upon the potential for male-female friendship formation, growth, and maintenance."[3] If this was true then of mere cross-sex friendships, it is doubly true now of cross-sex sexual friendships.

It is worth noting, too, that, as with cross-sex friends (but even more so here), if either or both sexual friends are in a romantic relationship with another person, problems with jealousy or other difficulties can easily occur. The reason for this is our cultural expectations for monogamous relationships, expectations that persist despite the high incidence of non-monogamy. (Studies suggest that 30–50 percent of men and 20–40 percent of women have had extramarital affairs.[4]) These expectations, which remain a dominant cultural ideal, are probably one of the major reasons why sexual friendships tend to occur among the single and unmarried.

Despite such limitations, sexual friendships are now a common occurrence, at least among American university students, which is where most of our knowledge of sexual friendships comes from. It has been suggested, however, that sexual friendships are a fact of life not only for many of these unmarried students, but also for those in their late teens and non-university students in their 20s and early 30s.[5] There is also evidence that sexual friendships are common among Canadian university students[6] and Swedish adolescents.[7] Further, my discussions with my students in the United Kingdom, Australia, and Denmark suggest that sexual friendships are also common in those countries. It also seems that sexual friendships play a role for older persons, especially women, who are coming out of a divorce, a situation in which such friendships might be more stable. After referring to the sexual friendships of some of her women clients, one divorce counselor says,

> while it may now be more socially acceptable for the younger generation to have a "friends with benefits" relationship, I think it's actually more likely to work when two emotionally intelligent, mature adults, with the skill set to negotiate safe sex and healthy emotional boundaries,

make the choice to limit their relationship to "FWB" while they focus on their children, career and personal growth, and healing.[8]

There are, however, various problems that face someone who wants to study these relationships. The first is to decide what counts as a sexual friendship. Although this might seem evident from the discussion so far, there is a lack of clarity among both the scholars who study the topic and those who are studied. One scholar, for example, refers to students who "hook up" with "one (or more) of their friends for casual loveless sex" for "the convenience of no-strings attached friends with benefits."[9] But this seems to be a confusion of casual sex or "hooking up," as it is called, with sexual friendship or the friends with benefits relationship. "Hooking up" is the current usual term for casual sex with acquaintances or strangers. As it is stated in one study, "Hookups are defined as a sexual encounter which may or may not include sexual intercourse, usually occurring on only one occasion between two people who are strangers or brief acquaintances."[10] This is quite distinct from sexual friendships. Studies show that sexual friends tend to participate in the same sorts of activities that nonsexual friends do.[11] This suggests that, as far as their friendship goes, they are not that distinct from close nonsexual friends.

Of course, with the advent of social media like Facebook, the word "friend" has acquired a new sense, a sense in which one can easily have 200 or more "friends," friends whom one does not even know. And it is true that some people use the term "friend with benefits" in this sort of loose way. The researcher Paul Mongeau and his co-workers, for example, suggest that there are seven types of friends with benefits relationships. These include relationships between "true friends," what they call "network opportunism," and "just sex," and then various transitional stages between these relationships and romantic relationships.[12] But as these researchers themselves say, the term "friend" in "friend with benefits relationship" is a misnomer when referring to a "just sex" relationship, for such relationships are essentially serial hook ups. Although the "network opportunism" relationship involves friends in a loose sense, the persons' association is based mainly on the fact that they are in the same network. They are not friends in the sense of having closeness and warmth or companionship. These relationships also typically seem to involve alcohol use.

It is only in the relationship of "true friends"—what Mongeau and his co-workers call a friend with benefit relationship in the traditional sense—that we find the normal idea of friendship. As one of the subjects in the study says when describing the meaning of the term "friend with benefits"—a subject who was in a "true friends" relationship—"It means someone who you know and care about as a friend/person who you also happen to have a sexual relationship with."[13] Note how the person here describes the friend as someone "who you also happen to have a sexual relationship with." This fits in well with what I said at the beginning of this chapter, namely, that the sexual part of such a relationship is an extra part of the relationship, rather than its main purpose. This sort of relationship is what I have been referring to as a sexual friendship. Therefore, sticking to this usual sense of the word "friend," it hardly seems correct to characterize the sex between friends as "casual." Friends have warm feelings and concern for each other. Calling the sex they have with each other "casual" seems to imply there are no such feelings or concern.

But what about calling their sex "loveless"? It is true that, not being in a romantic relationship, one could say their sex is "romantic-loveless." Yet romantic love is only one kind of love. There is also, for example, love in kinship: the love between mother and child, the love between brother and sister. There is also the love between friends. In the case of the love between friends, the word "love" would seem to refer to the warm feelings of care and concern that friends normally have toward each other. In this case, the sex that cross-sex friends have with each other is not loveless. Characterizing the sex that friends have with each other as "casual and loveless" is therefore wrong and seems little more than an attempt to disparage sexual friendships.

Other problems occur when people refer to these relationships, as they often do, as friendships that involve having sex but avoid the commitments and responsibilities that romantic relationships involve. It is true that sexual friendships do not normally involve these features of romantic relationships, but putting it like this seems to imply that a major purpose behind sexual friendships is the active avoidance of commitment and responsibility. Again, it is true that as the research shows, this is one of the reasons that some people have sexual friendships. But then, other people do not have this as a reason behind their sexual friendships. So here, too, it seems wrong to characterize sexual friendships as an avoidance of aspects of romantic love.

It is also worth noting that putting it this way makes it sound like romantic relationships are somehow the ideal relationship to which sexual friendships are an approximation (much like same-sex friendships are the ideal to which cross-sex friendships are an approximation). Rather than allowing that sexual friendships and romantic love are each relationships in their own right, this characterization implies that sexual friendships are deficient forms of romantic love. But there is no justification for seeing sexual friendships in this way. Many people in sexual friendships do not see their friendship like this. There is no desire to approximate a romantic relationship while avoiding the commitments that are sometimes (not always) part of romantic love. Rather, they simply enjoy each other's friendship and enjoy having sex with each other. Therefore, probably the best way to define sexual friendship is simply to say it is a relationship consisting of friends who have sex and do not see themselves as being romantic partners. The last clause is important since romantic partners can also be friends who have sex.

However, even with this definition in place, other problems remain. One is the conundrum of now finding out what exactly counts as having sex. For if one wants to distinguish between two types of friendship by pointing to the friends having sex in one of the friendships but not in the other, then one needs to know what counts as having sex. This difficulty of saying what counts as sex is something I already touched on in Chapter One. There I argued that it is difficult to draw a clear line between interactions that are not sexual and those that are. To be sure, at one end of the spectrum, some interactions, like shaking hands, are evidently not sexual interactions, while at the other end something like sexual intercourse clearly is a sexual interaction.

The problem comes, however, when we consider interactions like sensuous embracing, caressing of naked skin, and deep and passionate kissing. Are these sexual interactions or having sex? Earlier I argued that if someone tries to claim that such activities are not sexual because, say, they do not involve the genitals, then the implication is that other nongenital interactions are also not sexual. This would mean that a couple involved, for example, in a naked and passionate embrace with the man sucking on the woman's erect nipples and caressing her buttocks, while she holds his head firmly to her breast and fondles his thighs, were not engaged in a sexual interaction. Most people, however, would probably regard this interaction as clearly being sexual, even though the genitals are not involved. Even so, someone might feel that although this could be called a sexual interaction, it could not be called an instance of "having sex." For plainly, some people see the words "having sex" as referring only to sexual intercourse. But were we to accept this, we would then have to accept that homosexuals can never have sex with each other. This alone seems enough to reject the idea that "having sex" can only refer to sexual intercourse.

What, then, is it that determines whether an interaction is sexual? The answer to this, it should now be obvious, must be general enough to capture the wide variety of interactions that most people would consider to be sexual interactions. As I have argued elsewhere, what makes an interaction sexual is that it involves a mutual baring and caressing of naked skin, or at least that it aims in that direction.[14] One can, of course, attempt to sexually caress someone through his or her clothing. But normally the clothing is felt to be a barrier to the caress, since what the caress is really aiming at is the naked skin below the clothing. In those cases where the caress seems to be aiming specifically at the clothing, as in the case of someone with a clothing fetish, then the clothing, I would argue, has become a symbolic substitute for the naked skin. As a result, the natural object of the caress, though not naked skin itself, is still something that symbolizes the naked skin. Caressing, however, is something that can be done in various degrees and on various parts of the naked skin. This in turn implies that sexual interactions or having sex is also something that can be done in various degrees and in diverse ways.

With this idea established we are now in a better position to find the point where a cross-sex friendship moves over into a sexual friendship. For now it can be said that once cross-sex friends have engaged in a mutual baring and caressing of each other's naked skin, then a sexual interaction has taken place. Though, again, because of the possibility of degrees and places of caressing, some mutual baring and caressing might be seen as less of a sexual interaction than other instances. The difficulty of deciding when a cross-sex friendship becomes a sexual friendship is further exacerbated by the fact that, as we have seen, cross-sex friendships often already include hugging and flirtatious and sexual touching. And these interactions, if they involve mutual baring and caressing, are already sexual interactions.

It is not my intention to solve the problem of discovering the exact point where the one relationship changes into the other, and there may well be no exact point. The change could simply come as a matter of degree. If this is true, then what it shows is that many cross-sex friendships are not so distinct from sexual friendships. Nevertheless, it seems that most cross-sex friends will be able to agree on whether they have had sex or not, however they understand the idea of having sex. It is at this point where the friends have taken the first step to pass over into a sexual friendship.

But this is only the first step, for now another problem appears. This is the problem of deciding how many times cross-sex friends must have sex in order for their friendship to be considered a sexual friendship. The reason this is a difficulty is that we can easily imagine a case where a pair of long-term cross-sex friends who have never had sex suddenly find themselves having sex with each other. This could be for a variety of reasons: perhaps they were particularly close on that fateful afternoon, perhaps one of them felt especially lonely and embraced the other in a deep and passionate way, or perhaps alcohol loosened one or both of their inhibitions. But then we could imagine that on their next meeting both agreed, again for whatever reason, that their sexual encounter was a mistake that should not be repeated. Maybe one of them feels that if such encounters continued she might fall in love, and perhaps this is something she does not want. So, let us imagine that it does not get repeated. In circumstances like these, it seems that it would be wrong to say that these friends were now in a sexual friendship. This is because, even though they have had sex, their friendship has not become one in which sex is a feature of the friendship. Here it was merely a one-off thing. As a result, it does not continue to define the relationship.

But then how many times do friends have to have sex in order to be sexual friends? Again, there is no definite answer. Nevertheless, it seems to me that after a pair of friends have had sex on two occasions, sex is quickly becoming part of their friendship, for now it is no longer a one-off thing that will not happen again. It seems reasonable to say, therefore, that a cross-sex friendship has moved over into a sexual friendship after the friends have had sex at least two times. Even so, it might well be that a pair of friends have become sexual friends after just one instance of having sex. This is because maybe rather than having regretted their actions, they might well delight in this new aspect of their friendship and quickly make plans for the next time when they can have sex. If this is the case, then it would seem that they have entered a sexual friendship already after their first sexual encounter.

In addition to getting clear about what it is that makes up a sexual friendship, there is also the important issue of how sexual friends experience the quality of their friendship. For my purposes this is crucial because the quality of the relationship will affect the allure that takes place within the relationship. Therefore, in order to give an account of the allure that takes place in sexual friendships, one must first have an idea of how sexual friends experience the quality of the friendship. The reason this is an issue with sexual friendships and not so much with, say, cross-sex friendships, is that sexual friendships are contentious. Many people, including researchers in the area, have raised concerns about this trend in male–female relationships, pointing to various risks and possible negative features that such friendships can have. Even before the advent of large numbers of sexual friendships, one could find researchers expressing concern. In 1985 Lillian

B. Rubin, for example, cited several subjects from her study who expressed a negative view of mixing sex and friendship. Here are some of the views given by people she interviewed:

> "I don't think sex just inhibits friendship; it overpowers it and pushes it out."
>
> "Sex and friendship? Not a chance! Sex makes people possessive, which is exactly what friendships can't tolerate."
>
> "In my experience, and watching it with others, having a sexual relationship with someone seems most often to preclude the best part of a friendship—I mean the kind of trust and good will that goes with a good friendship."

In trying to explain these negative views about sexual friendship, Rubin considers the idea that society's norms around sex might be responsible. She ends up concluding, however, that the cultural mandates around sexuality and the way they affect us can only partly explain the difficulties most people have when they try to mix sex and friendship. For most of us, she says, the sexual encounter taps layers of feelings that, in adult life, are unique to it—feelings that are roused, at least in part, by the blurring of boundaries that take place only in sex. Whether in a man or a woman, this fusion seems to promise to fulfill our most archaic and infantile fantasies, exposing in us a set of needs and longings for union with another that are antithetical to friendship. For sex requires the merging of two people—not just physically but psychologically as well—where friendship rests on respect for separateness. Because of this, sexual friendships are most likely doomed to failure.[15]

With this conclusion it is clear that Rubin is not just citing her subjects' responses but is also supporting their views with arguments based on the nature of sexual interaction.

There are, however, difficulties with her argument, if for no other reason than that studies now show that the majority of sexual friendships are fairly successful. People in these relationships seem to mix sex and friendship at least as well as others mix sex and romantic love. Something must therefore be wrong with the argument she presents. And what is wrong, it seems to me, is that she has not given a good explanation of why the needs and longing for union in sexual interaction must be antithetical to friendship. The reason she gives for this is that sex requires a merging of two people while friendship requires a "respect for separateness." What this separateness refers to, I suppose, is a sense of being a distinct person and, consequently, within a friendship each person is required to respect the other's sense of being a distinct person. But I do not see why the merging felt while having sex cannot take place within a relationship in which each person also respects the other's sense of being a distinct person. Of course, when the two persons are having sex, they lose that sense of distinctness. But when they have finished having sex, they can regain their sense of being distinct persons and show respect for each other in this regard. Sexual friendships involve many things, including the sorts of activities and spending time together that are common in nonsexual friendships. When sexual friends are engaged in these activities, then plainly they can have a respect for separateness. When, however, they are engaged in sex, they can experience themselves as merging with indistinct boundaries.

One might be tempted to reply that the sense of merging experienced in sex is carried over into the nonsexual situation. For example, with a pair of lovers the sense of merging in sexual interaction might well have ripple effects that cross over into their nonsexual moments, thus sustaining a sense of blurred boundaries between each other even when they are not engaged in sex. It might do this, but must it necessarily or even normally do this? As long as we are considering romantic lovers, the argument has some plausibility. But what about sex between casual acquaintances or seen-before strangers? It seems unlikely that they will feel a sense of merging after they have had sex and run into each other on another occasion.

The reason why sexual activity might have these effects on nonsexual moments in a romantic relationship is that sexual interaction, or at least sexual desire, is an intimate part of romantic love, for to be romantically in love with someone implies having sexual desire for that person. However, romantic love is not part of sexual interaction or sexual desire. This is obvious from the fact that people can easily have sexual desire for or have sex with persons for whom they have no romantic desires. To be sure, having sex with someone might well lead to having romantic love toward that person. But then, it might just as well not lead to such desires.

Further, it must be noted that although the nonsexual features of friendship do not involve the sense of merging that sexual interaction does, they nevertheless involve another sense of merging. This is the attempt to overcome metaphysical isolation and become as close as possible to another awareness, which is the basis of all friendship. When this attempt to become as close as possible is engaged in by opposite-sex individuals who are also alluring to each other (that is, when they are cross-sex friends), then we have a relationship in which two senses of merging are taking place. Rather than being antithetical to each other, these two senses of merging seem instead to complement each other. This is because they both show, in their own ways, that strong bonds exist between the two persons. These are the bonds of sexual friendship.

Why, then, are negative views about sexual friendships so pervasive? A major impetus here, I would argue, is precisely those cultural norms that Rubin thinks are not enough to account for these ideas. For plainly, the idea of sexual friends goes against the West's traditional cultural norms. I mentioned in the last chapter the idea that cross-sex friends have a deviant and even threatening status. This is because they challenge traditional norms about men and women's relationships. The idea of sexual friendships, it would seem, challenges such norms even more. According to these norms, the only caring and kind relationship in which men and women should have sex is a romantic relationship. This view is well expressed by researcher Kathy Werking when she says that although friends may have sex, it "often signals the end of the 'friendship' and the beginning of a 'love relationship' since romance and sexuality are so closely aligned in romantic ideology."[16] The implication of this is that were people not under the sway of this ideology, then sex need not signal the end of a friendship nor the beginning of a love relationship.

That something like cultural norms or ideologies make people want to reject the idea of sexual friendship, rather than well-thought-out arguments about the nature of friendship or sexuality, is suggested also by the poor arguments that are often used. Examples of these can be found in the comments just cited from Rubin's study. Thus, one subject says, "I don't think sex just inhibits friendship; it overpowers it and pushes it out." But this cannot be true. If it were, then lovers could never be friends, for their sexual interactions would not only inhibit their friendship but would also overpower it and push it out. But as we know, many lovers are also friends.

In the second comment a subject argues that sex and friendship can never go together because "Sex makes people possessive, which is exactly what friendships can't tolerate." But if this were so, then casual acquaintances or strangers who have sex should also feel possessive of each other. But this is not usually the case. Moreover, there is also evidence that, far from being possessive, people involved in "hooking up" who might bump into each other on subsequent days (as on a university campus) will actively try to avoid each other after they have had sex.[17] We also know that sexual possessiveness or jealousy is closely related to feelings of low self-esteem. People with these feelings are more prone to jealousy than are those showing high self-esteem. Also, people in open or polyamorous relationships (love relationships with more than one partner) normally make agreements with each other about having multiple partners.[18] Here jealousy is infrequent. Finally, we know that jealousy is also much a function of cultural indoctrination, with some cultures, like traditional Polynesian culture or the polygamous Todas of India, showing little or no possessiveness or jealousy.[19] Consequently, there is no automatic connection between sex and possessiveness.

The last subject I cited says, "In my experience, and watching it with others, having a sexual relationship with someone seems most often to preclude the best part of a friendship—I mean the kind of trust and goodwill that goes with a good friendship." What this basically means is that you can never trust or have goodwill toward anyone you have sex with. If this were true, what a frightening world we would live in. Luckily, it is not true. Perhaps, however, the person means that it is only in friendship where sex has this peculiar effect. But if sex does not prevent trust and goodwill in love relationships, it seems implausible that it should do so in friendships.

There is also other evidence against these negative views of sex and friendship. One study from 2000 found that 67 percent of people who had sex with a friend felt that the sexual interaction had enriched their friendship.[20] In addition, other studies suggest that sexual friends not only engage in the same sort of activities as nonsexual friends do, but also show love, trust, and respect for each other, while seeing each other as important friends.[21] Further, the evidence suggests that even if the sexual interaction has stopped, which happens sometimes in sexual friendships, the majority of these relationships continue as friendships. Moreover, in about half of the friendships where sex has stopped, the friends report feeling just as close as or closer than they were earlier. In other words, the one-time sexual component of the friendship did not work to terminate the friendship or even damage the later nonsexual friendship.[22] As one woman said of her past sexual friendship, "THE BEST relationship I ever had was an FWB one. It lasted seven years. He is now married with a child and we still talk, no one ever knew about it. I think very fondly of him :) we had everything except the annoying expectations and 'ties'."[23]

Nevertheless, in addition to the positive aspects of sexual friendships, there are negative aspects. In another study researchers asked their subjects (university students) to identify possible risks with sexual friendships. The responses included the possibility of unreciprocated feelings, negative emotions, and damage to the friendship. Unfortunately, however, not all of the subjects had experiences with sexual friendships. It is therefore unclear how many of these responses come from direct experience with sexual friendship rather from discussions with others, speculation, or from previously held views.[24] In a further study, one involving Swedish late adolescents, hurt feelings, jealousy, and feelings of being exploited appeared when the development of romantic feelings was not reciprocated. This seems related to a common gender imbalance in expectations in sexual friendships, for it is more often the female who hopes the friendship will eventually become a romantic relationship. For females in this same study, there were also concerns about gossip and acquiring a bad reputation.[25] In addition, if a sexual friendship comes to an end, there can appear feelings of being deceived and a loss of being connected to social groups. These, however, seem to be more the case in those sexual friendships that emphasize the sexual aspect of the relationship rather than the friendship or nurturing aspects.[26]

The interesting thing, however, about these negative aspects of sexual friendships is that they do not sound terribly different from complaints raised in romantic love. Therefore, unreciprocated feelings, negative emotions, hurt feelings, jealousy, gender imbalances in expectations, and feelings of being exploited can all occur in romantic relationships. Consequently, if it is specifically these sorts of elements that lead someone to have a negative view of sexual friendships, then it seems that he or she should similarly have a negative view of romantic relationships. Of course, the person might feel that romantic relationships redeem themselves because romantic love is involved. But by the same token one could argue that sexual friendships redeem themselves because the love of friendship is involved.

The conclusion then seems to be that sexual friends, as I have been defining them, generally experience their relationships in a positive way. There is little evidence for claims about their involving risks, being emotionally damaging, or having other negative qualities that are not present in romantic relationships.

THE PLACE OF SEX IN SEXUAL FRIENDSHIP

I mentioned at the outset of this chapter that when cross-sex friends have sex, the relationship has altered in a basic way. The reason for this alteration is that in the moment of sexual contact, the result that sexual attraction was moving toward is at last achieved. This is because the final goal of sexual attraction is to bring one's own body into an intimate physical joining with the body of the sexually attractive person. Further, since sexual attraction is a basic motivation behind cross-sex friendships, once cross-sex friends have had sex, the reason for a basic motivation in the relationship has been achieved.

In a way, then, this event shakes the relationship to its core. For up to this juncture the person undergoing the attraction has never arrived at the point to which the attraction was leading her. The experience of her body intimately merged with the body of her friend existed in fantasy only. Of course, as mentioned, she will have known her friend's body well. She will have been near him, smelled him, seen him from up close, and probably hugged, kissed, and touched him. But the intimate sexual joining of her body with his always lay beyond all of this. That joining existed in her awareness as something her earlier touching and kissing were leading toward, but for which no concrete experience could be found. Then suddenly she is there! The physical body that had been attracting her abruptly envelops hers as she commingles in its form, losing her separateness.

This should not be taken to mean that sexual attraction terminates with the beginning of sex. For plainly the body of the attractive person retains its sexual attraction throughout the sexual engagement: people continue to embrace, caress, fondle, and kiss their partner's body while they have sex, continuing to find their partner's appearance, feel, taste, and smell sexually attractive. Still, a question could arise here concerning how the attraction could continue if the goal of the attraction has been achieved. The reply is that even though one is at last, say, locked in an embrace or in the midst of oral sex, one still feels the allure of one's partner drawing one onwards. Even though one has achieved an intimate merging with the other person's body through a particular caress, the allure of that person continues to impel one to repeat the caress or move on to a new caress, perhaps aiming at other attractive features of his or her body. This is because the experience of merging and losing separateness in sex is not a single-directional process that starts with separateness and ends with loss of separateness. It is rather a flickering in and out of merging, a blending and separating of bodies that move on to blend and separate again.

Interestingly enough, the movements and attempts to caress and hold the attractive person's body can here take on an almost automated quality, where the thrusting, clutching, and kneading seem nearly beyond the control of the person engaged in them. These actions can present themselves as being elicited from the attractive person's body where, say, his lips appear as "asking to be kissed" or her breasts as "begging to be held." For both men and women, this is a common way of describing their sexual experiences. But what is this sense of being drawn helplessly to grasp and merge with the attractive person's body? It is none other than the stuff of allure, allure continuing to work its magnetic powers in the throes of the sexual union.

It is also worth noting here that the end of a sexual interaction need not imply the end of sexual attraction. For people typically continue to find their partner as sexually attractive after having sex as before. In this situation a man, for example, after having had sex, may lean back against the pillows and, gazing at his partner's body, still find her smooth skin and curvaceous figure to be exquisitely attractive. The difference is that with the ending of the sexual interaction, especially if orgasm has taken place or there is a sense of completion to the sex act, the participants are typically physiologically spent with most tensions released. This gives sexual attraction (and also sexual desire) less of an urgency. The man in the example would still note the helplessness with which he feels drawn to his partner and still note the appearance of fantasies, but his relaxed state would enable him to watch these sensations from afar, as it were, without being swept away by them.

It is true that there is the well-known phenomenon of apparently losing sexual attraction for a partner immediately after having sex. In this sort of situation, commonly portrayed in films and literature, one of the partners gets up after having sex and, having apparently lost any interest in or attraction to the sexual partner, quickly gets dressed and slips out the door with a minimal goodbye. Or maybe he or she falls asleep after having sex and is able to wake early and slip away before his or her partner wakes up. There can, of course, be numerous reasons for such behavior. But one of the common explanations I have heard for at least some instances is that after having sex the person no longer finds the other sexually attractive and maybe even finds her unattractive. As a result, he just wants quickly to leave.

However, that a careful examination of most of these situations will probably reveal that sexual attraction did not really disappear. Instead, it was overwhelmed or smothered by contrary feelings, feelings that were able to come to the fore once the various tensions of the sex act subsided. These contrary feelings are typically those of shame, embarrassment, or guilt that some people feel over their own sexuality, typically a condition that their parents (who were also plagued by such shame, embarrassment, or guilt) drove into them at an early age. Some types of religion can also play a role in the creation and maintenance of these feelings and other negative views of sexuality. For people who have suffered this sort of treatment, such feelings, which were muted by the escalating sexual excitement, are then able to reassert themselves once the excitement begins to subside.

There is also often an element of self-deception here. For it is not always that the person simply did not know of his own feelings of embarrassment of guilt, but rather he chose to look the other way. He does this in order to achieve what he both deeply desires and also feels himself being relentlessly drawn toward, namely, a sexual union with his alluring partner. Once he has done this, he can then allow the feelings of embarrassment and guilt to return, for now it is too late for them to stop him. He can then safely indulge in these feelings and, leaving his partner immediately after having sex with her, try to convince himself that what he is doing is somehow equivalent to leaving her before he has had sex with her (at least it is still an instance of leaving her, he might think to himself, even if it is too late).

Note that, in none of this reaction did his partner's sexual attractiveness need to have disappeared for him. All that has changed is that the goal of allure has being achieved and the escalating sexual tensions of the sexual interaction have subsided.

The alteration that a cross-sex friendship undergoes once it involves sex is something that tends to remain regardless of how the relationship develops, whether the friends move on to incorporating more instances of sex while remaining friends, fall in love, or stop after one encounter. In all cases, having sex alters the friendship by achieving the goal of one of the basic motivations for the friendship, namely, the motivation of sexual attraction. Having sex is an event that fulfills a purpose on which the friendship was built. This would help explain why many people in sexual friendships feel that the sex has enriched their friendship. For the friendship, with its rudimentary element of sexual attraction, was always moving in this direction. But what sex with the friend would be like, what it would be like to hold the naked body in one's arms, to feel the moment of penetration or envelopment, and so on, all remained unknown.

It is true, as I mentioned, that cross-sex friends are in a better position to know what to expect sexually from each other than are strangers, but never having had sex with each other, there still exist uncertainties attached to these questions. Because sexual attraction lies at the nucleus of their friendship, a central element in their friendship gives rise to numerous uncertainties. With the having of sex, however, these uncertainties are suddenly replaced with concrete experience. This is the basis of the enrichment of the friendship, for the friendship is now enriched with intimate awareness of one's friend rather than surrounded by uncertainties. The intimate awareness here is sexual awareness. Upon having sex with one's friend, one comes to know him or her in a deep and familiar way, for in sexual interaction, façades are difficult to maintain. Naked and exposed, we present ourselves to the eyes, hands, and body of another individual. How we present ourselves and the look and feel of our body is immediately revealed to our partner.

A pivotal event in this act of revealing is the removal of clothing. I earlier mentioned that clothing plays a major role in enhancing sexual attraction. One of the reasons for this is that clothing can accentuate and draw attention to various aspects of the body while nevertheless hiding them. In this situation the person under the sway of the sexual attraction will be brought to fantasize about what those accentuated but hidden parts of the body would look like once the barrier of clothing is removed. Therefore, as long as someone is clothed, just what these concealed parts of the body look like to others remain in the realm of fantasy.

Once the clothing comes off, however, fantasy about what the body looks and feels like gives way to reality. The control that the clothing maintained is gone, and the body is presented for what it is. In such circumstances the naked individual is suddenly vulnerable to the partner because he or she has lost that measure of control that clothing afforded. Vulnerability also appears in the form of being vulnerable to the partner's touch; being naked before one's partner exposes the body to whatever sort of handling, caress, or fondling the partner may do. Even in those situations where individuals have sex partially clothed, hands still make their way under the clothing or, in sexual intercourse, the penis is exposed to the caresses of the vagina and the vagina to the caresses of the penis. The individual is also vulnerable because as the individual enters the sex act, controlled or calculated responses become more and more difficult to maintain as one melts with desire, as it were, under the caresses of one's partner.

As I have argued in *The Nature of Sexual Desire* these instances of being vulnerable before one's partner while having one's partner vulnerable before oneself are the heart of the experience of sexual interaction. We put ourselves in this vulnerable situation before our partner in order that our partner may respond with care, for to be vulnerable is to be in need of care. In sexual interaction this is expressed in the form of baring and caressing. Thus, in baring one's body one becomes vulnerable, and in having one's naked body caressed one is taken care of. The caress takes care of the individual because the individual's reason for baring her body was in order that she might be caressed. And these warm and intimate acts of baring and caressing are precisely the goal of sexual attraction. They are what sexual attraction is ultimately drawing us toward.

It can now be seen why having sex together enables cross-sex friends to know each other in a deep and intimate way. For in having sex with each other, they expose these vulnerabilities to each other. And in experiencing and learning each other's vulnerabilities, they come to know each other in an especially close way. Moreover, they respond to each other's vulnerabilities by caressing each other, thus showing mutual care. I just mentioned that the friendship is enriched with the friends' intimate awareness of each other. Here, then, we come to a more specific account of how the friendship is thus enriched, namely, through an awareness of each other's vulnerabilities and how to show care for those vulnerabilities. In other words, it is enriched by an awareness of each other's naked bodies and how to caress each other's body.

Because this sexual connection enables the friends to know each other deeply and intimately, it is natural to wonder how the sex they have can be considered an addition to the friendship. For it seems that an element that leads to this sort of experience would have won a central place in the friendship. The way of understanding this, I think, is not to forget that the friendship is already a powerful tie between the two individuals. The sharing of personal information, the emotional support, care and concern, and companionship, work without the help of sexual interaction to forge strong bonds between the friends. Furthermore, there is also the powerful tie of sexual attraction even before there was any sex. To be sure, the friends' sexual interaction is a direct result of their mutual sexual attraction, but the attraction exists whether or not it comes to fruition in sexual interaction. Consequently, when sex arrives on the scene, it is as an extra addition to the already existing bonds of friendship and sexual attraction. It is in this sense that sex in a sexual friendship is an addition to the relationship rather than its essential purpose or core.

There is, however, the possibility for a man and woman to meet in, say, a hookup-like situation, have sex, and then later become sexual friends while continuing to have sex. In this case the sex is not something extra that is added to an already established cross-sex friendship, rather it is a basic element in the relationship straight from the start. Here, sex might not appear to be something additional to the friendship.

It is definitely true that there are sexual friendships that start this way, though my guess would be that they are far less common than those that begin with friendship and then progress to sexual friendship. Nevertheless, the decisive point is not whether sex came before or after the friendship was formed but what role the sex plays in the relationship. If the relationship is one that emphasizes the friendship over the sex, then whether or not sex came first, it is a sexual friendship. If sex eclipses the well-wishing, well-doing, and enjoyment of just being together, then it seems the relationship is not properly called a sexual friendship. Rather, it would seem to be more of a serial hookup.

However, even in the case of a true sexual friendship, there is no guarantee that things will not change. The sex in their friendship might rise to prominence, usurping the role of the friendship. We have seen that there are "just sex" relationships or sexual friendships that stress the sexual aspect of the relationship rather than the nurturing aspects of friendship. It might well be that some of these relationships were originally "true friends," sexual friendships that eventually transmuted into more of a mainly sexual relationship. In such cases sex would not be an extra element in the relationship, but then the relationship would no longer be what I have been referring to as a sexual friendship.

Because sex allows cross-sex friends to know each other in this way, a relation between sex and friendship is immediately visible. Friendship, as we have seen, is based on the attempt to come as close as possible to another person's awarenesses. But sexual interaction shares a similar feature, for it, too, is an attempt to get as close as possible to another person, though here it is the other person's body rather than his or her awareness that one is seeking to get close to. In friendship the effort to achieve this closeness stems ultimately from the attempt to overcome metaphysical isolation. Could it be that in sexual interaction the effort to achieve the bodily closeness stems from a similar attempt to overcome a form of isolation?

The answer is forthcoming when we notice that the sex engaged in by cross-sex sexual friends is sex between two people of different sexes or genders, namely a male and a female. For what a male lacks in terms of gender is femaleness and what a female similarly lacks is maleness. In other words, a male is isolated from the experience of being a female by the fact that he is a male. Conversely, a female is isolated from the experience of being a male by the fact that she is a female. Because of this, the sex between cross-sex friends can be seen as a way of breaking out of this gender isolation, as it might be called, by getting as close as possible to the body of the opposite sex. This is why having sex often involves acts of bodily penetration or envelopment. For in performing acts like sexual intercourse, fellatio, sucking on a breast, inserting fingers into the vagina or anus, pressing the tongue into an ear, or deep kissing with the tongue, one is either entering the body of another person or taking the body of another person into one's own. By entering or being entered, one is actually mixing one's body with another's body. This is especially so when bodily fluids like saliva, sperm, and vaginal secretions, which are part of one person's body, are taken into the other person's body.

It might be felt, however, that this view of sexual interaction is called into question by the existence of homosexual interaction. For homosexual partners are of the same gender and so not isolated from their partner's gender. I think, however, at the subjective level of experience (which is also what I am discussing with heterosexuals), there is a sense in which homosexuals also undergo a sense of isolation from their own gender. This is why they engage the same gender sexually, namely, to have a deeper access to their own gender. I have discussed this process elsewhere and so will not pursue it further here.

It is in this mixing, then, that one at last acquires a sense of having broken out of gender isolation by mixing one's body with a body of the attractive gender. Here the man finds his maleness diffusing into and being absorbed by his partner's femaleness, while the woman feels her femaleness diffusing into and being absorbed by her partner's maleness. And, similarly, the man feels his partner's femaleness diffusing into and being absorbed by his maleness, while the woman feels her partner's maleness diffusing into and being absorbed by her femaleness. In sexual intercourse, for example, both the man and woman can feel their sex organs merging indistinctly into the partner's sex organs, where the perimeters of the penis and the walls of the vagina lose their distinctness and seem to commingle.

Similar experiences of merging with the opposite gender appear in other types of sex acts, though each with its own variation. A good account of this experience in performing fellatio, and how it differs from sexual intercourse, is given by Catherine Millet in her autobiography *The Sexual Life of Catherine M.* Here she says,

> there is an obscure identification with the member you appropriate. During an exploration carried out simultaneously with fingers and tongue you come to know every last detail of its topography and even its tiniest reactions—perhaps better than its owner. As a result there is a feeling of ineffable mastery: a tiny quivering of the end of the tongue, and you unleash a disproportionate response. Added to this is the fact that taking something right into your mouth gives you a more thorough feeling of being filled than when it is the vagina that is occupied. The feeling in the vagina is diffuse, radiating outwards, the occupant seems to melt there, whereas you can perfectly distinguish the gentle proddings of the glans with the inside or outside of the lips, on the tongue, the palate and even in the throat. Not to mention the fact that, in the final phase, you taste the sperm. In short, you are touched as subtly as you yourself touch.[27]

We are thus given a detailed account of merging with the opposite gender from the female point of view in two distinct sex acts. In sexual intercourse, Millet describes her experience of the penis seeming to melt within her vagina, while in fellatio she identifies with her partner's penis by discerning its movements through contact with the various parts of her mouth, provoking responses with her tongue, and coming to know intimately its structure through her exploration with both her fingers and her mouth. All of this leads her to feel that she might know the penis even better than its owner. In a sense, then, her partner's penis becomes hers. This identification is further aided by knowing the taste of the sperm. The touching of her partner by her is, at the same time, a touching of her by him, a touching that underlies a female's obscure identification with a male's penis. This is an overcoming of gender isolation.

It is significant to note that a similar idea is also expressed in the ancient Chinese sex manuals. Here, in sexual intercourse, the man and woman are seen to exchange their male and female essences. This is done through the sperm of the man entering the woman and being absorbed by her, and the vaginal secretions of the woman entering the man by being absorbed by his penis. This is an exchange of the female's yin and the male's yang, two primal forces in ancient Taoist philosophy.[28] This is another way of expressing the loss of gender isolation that transpires in sexual interaction. In this way one feels that one's gender has been completed by something that it lacked, namely, the opposite gender. (Homosexual interaction involves a similar mechanism, but here the person feels himself or herself completed by diffusing into and being absorbed by another instance of his or her own gender.)

The view that sexual interaction is an attempt to somehow absorb the other gender into oneself is naturally dependent on a further idea. This is the idea that the gender of the attractive individual is an important aspect of what one is attracted to or of what one desires. My view that it is of crucial significance has, however, been criticized by the psychologist Meg Barker. Barker states that what I say goes against "the reported lived experience of many who identify as bisexual and who state that they are attracted to others 'regardless of gender' or find other aspects of sex more important than gender (such as the sexual practice engaged in, or who is active or passive)."[29]

Unfortunately, however, she gives no data to support her claim. There might well be individuals who fit these descriptions, though even here I would first have to know of any fantasies or symbolism that attend the sexual practices before I would rule out gender as playing a significant role. But even if there were such individuals, they would clearly not be typical. The available research suggests that for the majority of bisexuals, gender is a significant factor in sexual attraction. In *Dual attraction: Understanding bisexuality*, which is a major study based on numerous interviews with bisexual men and women (that is, on their lived experiences), the authors summarize the results of the interviews by saying, "Each gender was said to have something unique or different to offer, which formed the basis of bisexuals' dual attractions."[30] This makes it plain that gender is indeed the basis of bisexual attraction and that the majority of bisexuals are not attracted to others "regardless of gender." In this way bisexual attraction has the same basis as heterosexual or homosexual attraction; it is just that they are sexually attracted to both genders.

Coming back now to the idea of bodily penetration or envelopment, it is difficult to draw a clear distinction between sexual acts that are instances of this and sexual acts that are not. If someone who is naked embraces another person who is naked, wrapping his or her arms and legs around that person, then there is a clear sense in which his or her body is receiving and enveloping the other person's body, naked skin against naked skin. But this is not altogether distinct from what happens in sexual intercourse. Here the woman's vagina takes in and envelops the man's penis, again with naked skin against naked skin. Therefore, were a man to be embracing a woman while she at the same time was taking his penis into her vagina, then there is also a clear sense in which their bodies are involved in interpenetration. This would seem even more so if the woman's tongue or breast were, at the same time, in the man's mouth. Here we have a good example of the mixing of bodies, an event in which the man and woman lose their distinctness and acquire the sense of merging their genders together. Again, I have discussed these issues in-depth elsewhere. For my present purposes it is merely important to see that in these acts of entering or incorporation, an individual has brought his or her body, in one of the closest ways possible, together with the body of another person.

In this way sexual friends clearly have two paths to mutual closeness, namely, the path of friendship and the path of sexual interaction. Further, these paths do not seem fully independent from each other. This is indicated by the fact that a majority of sexual friends report that having sex with each other has enriched their friendship and made them feel closer. This suggests that having sex has made them feel closer as friends. Although there are no data here, it seems reasonable to suppose that being friends would affect the closeness they also feel as sexual partners. For knowing and caring about each other as friends would seem to have a positive influence on their sexual interactions. If one knows one's sexual partner well and has care and concern for him or her, then one will most likely take time and effort, while using one's intimate knowledge, to tend to his or her sexual needs.

It seems significant to note that in having two paths to closeness, sexual friends have twice as many such paths as same-sex friends do. For sexual friends have both friendship and sex as ways to enrich their friendship and bring them closer together, while same-sex friends have only friendship. Further, since sexual friends tend to engage in the same sort of friendship exchanges and activities that same-sex friends do, it does not seem that same-sex friendships have any basic features that are lacking in sexual friendships. That is, it does not look like same-sex friendships have a further way for achieving closeness that is lacking in sexual friendships. The intimacy of women's same-sex friendships and the shared activities of men's same-sex friendships can both be found in sexual friendships.

It is true that same-sex friends can share and discuss various sorts of personal experiences that sexual friends cannot. For example, two men friends can exchange personal experiences they have had in their relationships as men with female romantic partners. Or two women friends can share their experiences of pregnancy with each other. These sorts of shared experiences are ones that sexual friends, being opposite sexes, cannot engage in. Sexual friends cannot share experiences they have both had as men, for only one of them is a man. Similarly, sexual friends could never both share their experiences of pregnancy, for only the woman could ever have been pregnant.

Still, I am not so sure that these sorts of "dependent on being the same sex" exchanges represent a distinct path to intimacy and closeness that is necessarily lacking in sexual friendships. Any friends, whether same-sex or cross-sex, will have similar experiences that they share with each other. Two cross-sex sexual friends, for example, might both have done postgraduate work in mathematics, worked in the same restaurant, or traveled up the Amazon. Their discussions of these experiences will not depend on their both being the same sex; whether or not they are the same sex, they can still have both engaged in these sorts of activities. But their discussions will, however, depend on their both, for example, having traveled up the Amazon. It is not obvious that sharing experiences that only people of the same sex can share represents a special way of gaining closeness that is not found in other sorts of intimate sharing that are available to sexual friends.

Because same-sex friendships lack the sexual component of sexual friendships, a natural thought here might be that they avoid problems that might come along with a sexual relationship: jealousy, possessiveness, unreciprocated feelings, and various other experiences that might lead to a rupture in closeness. However, as we have seen, the evidence does not support the idea that such issues occur in any frequency in sexual friendships. It is true that people in sexual friendships can develop these problems. But this mainly seems to be when one partner has romantic expectations that the other partner has not. In these cases, a lack of open communication about the nature of the relationship, rather than the sexual interaction, seems to be the heart of the problem.

Moreover, even if same-sex friendships do avoid problems that might come along with a sexual relationship, they do not have a monopoly on avoiding problems. For sexual friendships, being cross-sex friendships, avoid the rivalry, competition, and jealousy that can appear in both male and female sex friendships. So, what same-sex friendships gain in avoiding one sort of problem, they lose in ushering in another. That is, it is not evident that same-sex friendships are ahead of sexual friendships in avoiding problems.

The view that sexual friendships might have an extra path to intimacy and mutual closeness that is lacking in same-sex friendships is naturally controversial view. The reason is it challenges the commonly held view that same-sex friendships are the ideal or authentic friendships. For here we have another sort of friendship—a sexual friendship—that seems to have a further way of achieving central elements in friendship, a way denied to same-sex friendships. This raises the intriguing possibility that it is same-sex friendships that may be lacking in closeness, at least compared to sexual friendships.

Further, since even cross-sex friendships without sex still have sexual attraction, and since sexual attraction can lead people to have sex, then cross-sex friendships at least have the possibility for achieving the sort of closeness gained in sexual friendships. Same-sex heterosexual friendships, because they are heterosexual, do not have this possibility. And even if there were heterosexual same-sex friends who came up with the idea of having sex in order increase their intimacy, such a plan would be doomed from the start because it would not be driven by sexual attraction or sexual desire. That is, it would involve neither the experience of allure nor the desires to be naked and vulnerable before each other in order to be cared for by a caress. It would therefore be contrived and consequently fail to achieve genuine intimacy.

Interestingly enough, something similar would seem to be true in same-sex homosexual friendships, for as we have seen, sexual attraction seems to be lacking in these friendships. Moreover, when male homosexuals want emotional closeness and support, they typically turn to their female friends, not their male friends. But because of the man's homosexuality, these friendships with females are lacking in sexual attraction and, accordingly, in the possibility of genuine sexual interaction. This does seem to put sexual friendships in the unique position of being able to achieve an enhanced degree of closeness and intimacy that is lacking in other sorts of friendships.

The obvious way of resisting this conclusion is to claim that having sex does not give the sort of closeness and intimacy that is the stuff of friendship. Friendship is about mutual liking, psychological and emotional closeness, and companionship, it could be said, and the fondling, caressing, and nakedness of sexual interaction have little to do with these ties of friendship.

I do not, however, see what sort of argument could support such a claim. It is obviously true that people can have sex without being friends, but this does not mean that sex cannot, in other circumstances, be an element in achieving deeper levels of friendship. This can be seen by reflecting over other elements in friendship and how the same holds true for them. Shared activities, for example, also can be engaged in without the participants' being friends. But, similarly, this does not mean that shared activities, in other circumstances, cannot be an element in achieving deeper levels of friendship. Further, it is also true that a man and woman can be friends without having sex. But again, this does not show that sex cannot play a role in friendship. This, too, is supported by the fact that the same is true of other elements of friendship. For example, people can be friends without sharing intimate details of their lives. But here, too, this does not imply that sharing such details cannot, under different conditions, help to make a friendship stronger.

All of this merely shows it is possible that sex can lead to the sort of intimacy and closeness that is part of friendship. What shows that it is actual are the experiences of those in sexual friendships who report that having sex with their cross-sex friend has enriched their friendship and brought them closer together. Further, it is not just sexual friends who are brought closer by having sex, for the same is true of romantic partners. But this is something I will come to in the next chapter. For now let us turn to the nature of the allure that exists between sexual friends.

THE ALLURE OF SEXUAL FRIENDS

This is an area where, unfortunately, there has been little research. Not only has the study into sexual friendships themselves been minimal, but the study of sexual attraction in these relationships, and thus the way in which sexual friends undergo allure toward each other, has been all but ignored. In my own discussions with my students and other people, however, I have been able to come up with an overview of the process.

The first thing to notice is that, just as with the allure of a cross-sex friend, the allure of a sexual friend is something that takes place within the context of friendship. Therefore, the friendship provides a warm and protective environment in which the experience of allure unfolds. The mutual liking of sexual friendship draws the friends together and so works to support the allure that is also taking place. Because it is a sexual friendship, there is another powerful element added to this mixture. For here the person appears in the other friend's awareness as a friend with whom he or she has nakedly caressed. Therefore, with a sexual friend the goal of the allure felt toward the cross-sex friend has become realized. This is potent because it has given the person a taste of what her allure for her friend has always been drawing her toward.

In a way, the allure of the sexual friend can be said to have validated itself in the caresses exchanged with the friend. It demonstrated that it was capable of bringing about the state of affairs it had been working toward. In the case of a stranger, the allure draws one on to something unknown. In the case of a cross-sex friend, the allure has more concrete material at its disposal, giving the goal of allure—an intimate baring and caressing—the sense of potential attainability. But what this would be like if it were attained remains in the end unknown. With a sexual friend, however, this potential attainability turns into actual attainability. One has been brought to the ultimate goal of allure, namely, intimately joining and mixing bodies with one's alluring friend. The sexual encounters with one's friend then remain in one's awareness to become an important content of the allure, displaying clearly what the allure of one's sexual friend is alluring one toward. It is almost as if the experience of allure is saying to the individual under its sway, "See! Here is what awaits you at the end of this magnetic journey, and you know this is true because you have been here before."

Now, it will be recalled from the last chapter that although cross-sex friendship and allure are separate, the friendship nevertheless blends with and affects the allure. It does this much like the background of a portrait blends with and affects our perception of the image in the foreground. This same relation between the friendship and allure also holds for sexual friendship and the allure that is felt for a sexual friend. In the case of sexual friendship, however, the friendship that affects the allure is a more complicated friendship. This is because, in addition to being cross-sex friends, the friends are also sexual partners. Thus, they already have what cross-sex friends have but, in addition, they also have a sexual relationship. This is a further dimension that, because of the prior experience of having sex with one's friend, and because of the exposure of vulnerabilities inherent in sexual interaction, will bring various complexities with it. This in turn means that the friendship will tend to affect the allure felt toward a sexual friend in a more complex way than it does with the allure felt toward a cross-sex friend.

To see how the complexity of sexual friendship affects the allure of the sexual friend, imagine the case of a man meeting his sexual friend. When he sees her coming to greet him, she is not presented to his awareness as an individual who has two distinct relationships with him. That is, he does not experience her as a friend on one hand and a sexual partner on the other. Rather, he experiences these two aspects of her relationship to him as deeply interwoven and inseparable. She is a sexual friend, and neither of these two aspects of their relationship enters his awareness of her without the other. For example, let us say that as she approaches him she gives him a warm smile and begins to quicken her pace toward him. These are the signs of her friendship. But these signs of friendship do not appear unattached from signs of other aspects of her relationship to him. Thus, the smile of friendship she gives him comes from the same eyes that, he can well remember, closed heavily when he last took off her clothes and from the same mouth that kissed him deeply as he embraced her naked body. Likewise, the legs that quicken her steps toward him, showing her desire for and enjoyment of his company, are the same legs that earlier wrapped around him when they last had sexual intercourse. In this way, and numerous others, his awareness of her friendship with him is infiltrated with his awareness of her sexual partnership with him. Let us now see how this works on the elements of allure.

Using the same example, it is not difficult to imagine that as the man sees his sexual friend approaching him, he is immediately overtaken by her allure. The shortness of her steps, the sway of her hips, and the fluttering of her hair in the wind all come together to grip him like the field of a magnet, creating the sense of being drawn helplessly toward her. But here, too, in the same moment that she allures him with her physical appearance, she also presents herself as a friend—and not just a friend, but as a friend who is at the same time a sexual partner. This friendship and sexual partnership are experienced, as I have argued, as deeply interwoven and always together. However, for the purposes of revealing the allure of the sexual friend, one can nevertheless focus in turn on each individual aspect. Focusing on the friendship in this way, it will be seen that, as in a cross-sex friendship, the friendship here is also a form of attraction, an attraction that ultimately has its roots in the attempt to overcome metaphysical isolation by coming as close as possible to another consciousness. This attempt finds its expression here as happiness and mutual liking with its well-wishing, well-doing, and pure enjoyment in each other's company, experiences that make friends continue to seek each other out. Therefore, it works in unison with the pull of allure, providing a warm and supportive context for allure to take place.

In the case of a sexual friendship, however, the friend is also at the same time a sexual partner. This means that with the allure of a sexual friend, the goal of allure—sexual interaction—has already been achieved. This affects the allure in a basic way, for now the goal of allure is known with full clarity. Here one knows exactly what such an intimate joining will involve, a knowledge that creates a clear picture of the goal that is promptly taken up and set to work within the experience of allure.

To be sure, there might well be variations according to the sort of sexual interaction, the surroundings, or the state of the sexual partners, but the general sense of what it is to have sex with that particular person will tend to remain the same. This has an important effect on the pull of the allure. For in having been allured to having sex with one's friend before, one knows full well what one is being allured to the next time. The subsequent experience of the pull of one's friend's allure will therefore tend to present itself to awareness in a more focused and clarified way. This is a focus and clarity that can only come with knowing by direct acquaintance the sensations of baring and caressing that awaits one as the goal of allure. With an alluring stranger, and even with a cross-sex friend (as I have been defining them), there has been no previous sexual interaction. This gives the sense of being drawn less of a sharpness and lucidity about where exactly one is being drawn to. One is being drawn, one knows, to an intimate physical connection with the alluring person, but what specifically will happen, what it will feel like, remains unknown. Hence the awareness of being drawn will, in these sorts of cases, tend to lack the directional sharpness, as it might be called, that is more at home with the allure of the sexual friend. When we bring this together with the attraction of friendship, we then have a sharp and lucid sense of being swept along in a definite direction amid a warm and supportive current. This is the experience of being drawn in allure toward one's sexual friend.

Turning now to the element of helplessness in allure, here, too, it is obvious that the sexual friendship will have an effect. The main reason for this is that just as there is a sense of helplessness in sexual attraction, so is there a sense of helplessness in sexual interaction. In sexual attraction, helplessness appears in the experience of allure. It is the sense that one is being drawn beyond one's will toward sexual contact with the attractive person. In sexual interaction the sense of helplessness appears at several places. I already mentioned that in the midst of having sex the various activities of grasping, holding, and thrusting can take on a nearly automated quality. In these instances, such actions seem to proceed more and more of their own accord as the excitement escalates and we are swept along in a delirium of desire. Freud, for example, refers to the compelling aspect of what he calls fore-pleasure.[31] This is the erotic pleasure that arises in the buildup of the tension leading toward orgasm. It is a pleasure that seems to compel one to continue increasing the tension in the sexual act. The universality of this experience is suggested by a similar reference in writings from ancient India. Vātsyāyana refers to this in the *Kāma Sūtra* as "making furious love" and compares someone in this state to "a speed-maddened horse, flying at a gallop and seeing neither holes nor ditches."[32] A person in this situation is, in an obvious sense, helpless, for she seems to have lost something of the control over her actions. Plainly, she is not completely out of control but has rather got herself into a state where her actions require minimal effort to continue and maximum effort to stop. This creates the sensation of being helpless to stop.

This is connected to further instances of helplessness that can appear in sexual interaction. One instance is the point at which the rising tensions of fore-pleasure suddenly give way to a sense of the inevitability of orgasm along with an accompanying concentration of erotic pleasure. Peak pleasure, as I call it, is the abrupt and rapid ascension of pleasure to its highest point. Here, one genuinely is out of control as one feels involuntarily catapulted upward to the highest point of tension and the highest intensity of pleasure. For the male, this also carries with it an awareness of the inevitability of ejaculation. Reaching this distant point, suddenly there is an instantaneous bursting of all the tensions as one is thrown back and downward onto waves of pulsation (here is where the male's ejaculation occurs).

Also, in the moment of bursting, peak pleasure suddenly fragments, disappearing into the distance, only to be immediately replaced by a pleasure of release as one is carried out on waves of contractions. For the female, with her distinct ability for multiple orgasms, this sequence has the possibility of repeating itself, though here the pleasure of release is hardly allowed to show itself before the next rush to peak pleasure sets in. (Multiple orgasms—repetitive appearances of peak pleasure—are possible for males.[33]) All of this, from the moment peak pleasure sets in, is virtually beyond voluntary control. Accordingly, the sense of helplessness is a constant feature of this sequence of sexual interaction.

Here, then, is the connection to vulnerability. For at the same time one is helpless, one is also vulnerable. And vulnerability, as I have tried to show, is a fundamental element in sexual interaction. To bare one's body to another person is to be vulnerable to him or her in various ways. One has lost control over the other person's perceptions of one's body. One is thus helpless before the other person's gaze as one's body is presented to him or her fully revealed. One is also helpless in a sense before the other person's touch, for there is no protective barrier of clothing between the other person's skin and one's own. One could even say that in sexual intercourse, as the penis and vagina are brought together, the vagina is helpless to stop the penetration of the penis, which in turn is helpless to stop being enveloped by the vagina. Obviously, one can intervene here with hands or various bodily movements, or the man could try to distract himself in order to prevent or lose an erection (and thus envelopment by the vagina), just as the woman could try to bring on a case of vaginismus or sealing off of the vaginal entrance (which cannot be done voluntarily anyway). But the excited sex organs themselves are incapable of preventing their union and thus helpless before each other.

Because the sense of helplessness is closely connected to sexual interaction, it is understandable how this experience is no stranger to those in a sexual friendship, for a definitive feature of this sort of friendship is that it involves sexual interaction. Consequently, the element of helplessness in allure finds a natural companion in the helplessness of sexual interaction. How, then, does the helplessness of sexual interaction affect the helplessness of allure? To answer this, it must be remembered that when someone is under the allure of his sexual friend, somewhere in his mind are the memories of their earlier sexual interactions. In other words, not only is the individual aware of the helplessness that his sexual friend's allure is casting over him, he is also aware of the helplessness that transpired in their earlier instances of having sex.

I am not saying that the awareness of helplessness during sex will necessarily be at the forefront of his mind, but only that when he comes under the allure of his friend, there will tend to be a vague sense of it. For not only is this an evident feature of sexual interaction, but both helplessness and an image of sexual interaction (here based on actual experiences with the friend) are also central features of allure. Therefore, in the very moment that he is aware of his helplessness under the allure of his sexual friend, he is simultaneously aware of the helplessness in his sexual interactions with her. Thus, there will be an intensified prominence of the element of helplessness, for the experience of helplessness doubles its appearance in the allure of a sexual friend.

Although the experience of being drawn helplessly toward one's friend occurs in sexual friendships, it only does so as part of the allure. As just mentioned, its position is intensified due to the experiences of having had sex with one's alluring friend, experiences that involved other instances of helplessness. Still, these other instances of helplessness, which occurred during sexual interaction, share much in common with the alluring experience of being helplessly drawn. As a result, the memories of helplessness experienced during sex with one's friend are easily merged in awareness with the experience of being helplessly drawn. That is, they become essentially part of the helplessness component of allure.

This is a distinction between the allure of the cross-sex friend and the allure of the sexual friend. For in cross-sex friendships the friends have not had sex and so will not have experienced helplessness while having sex with each other. (Again, however, it must be remembered there is no hard and fast line between what counts as having sex and what does not. And since cross-sex friends typically engage in extensive mutual touching, such an interaction may well come close enough to being an instance of having sex. This, in turn, might well bring with it the experience of helplessness.) Because of this, it is evident that the sexual part of a sexual friendship—namely, the having of sex—has an influence on the helplessness experienced in the allure of the sexual friend. But what about the friendship part of a sexual friendship? Does it, too, have an influence here?

At first glance, this might not seem to be the case. For if we look at the attraction of friendship, what we will tend to see is mutual liking, trust, loyalty, and so forth. There is nothing in the attraction of friendship per se that suggests an ever-present component of helplessly being drawn. Nevertheless, the experience of helplessness itself, as opposed to being helplessly drawn, is something that makes an appearance in friendship. As we have seen, caring for one's friend is a common feature of friendship. This seems related to the basic features of well-wishing and well-doing. For to wish someone well and to do what one can to bring about that wellness is to care about the person. One can care about a person who is in any condition, but caring about someone who is helpless seems an especially appropriate use of care.

In this way, the awareness of helplessness is something that can easily enter the experience of friendship. Therefore, the allure of one's sexual friend and the attraction one has for her as a friend are yet again linked by a common feature, namely, the feature of helplessness. In the case of allure, the feature of helplessness appears in the awareness of being helplessly drawn, while in the case of friendship it appears in the awareness of caring for or being cared for by one's friend. In the case of friendship, however, it is not an ever-present feature as it is in allure. In friendship it is mostly a possibility that one, as a friend, wants to be vigilant about. Were one's friend to suddenly be in need of help, one would want to be available to provide such help. Still, it is enough to help establish a connection in one's awareness between the friendship one has with one's sexual friend and the allure one has for her. The route for this connection is simply that in having allure for my sexual friend, I am aware of being helplessly drawn toward her as my sexual partner. But since she is also my friend, I am at the same time aware that she cares for me, and especially so when I am helpless. Consequently, although I am helplessly drawn toward her, I can rest assured that she will care for me.

Throughout the discussion so far, I have been referring to such things as a clear picture of the goal, an image, or a memory of the sexual union of the sexual friends. What all of these terms refer to, as should now be plain, is the brief sexual fantasy that is the third element of allure. The fact that it has been impossible to discuss fully the other two elements—the sense of being drawn and the experience of helplessness at being thus drawn—without likewise mentioning the fantasy element shows the essential interconnectedness of these elements. But is there a connection between sexual friendship and the element of sexual fantasy in allure? I have already shown that sexual friendship has an influence on the other two elements of allure. It therefore seems likely that the sexual friendship will similarly have an influence on the element of sexual fantasy.

That this is what happens is easily seen when we recall the typical origin of sexual fantasies. For sexual fantasies, as has been noted, tend to be firmly tied to reality, typically being about past or current sexual partners and specific sexual acts. This is especially so for the brief fantasies of allure. For when one is under another person's allure, what one is allured to is a sexual joining with *that* person's body. It is therefore an image of an intimate joining of one's own body with that particular person's body that is the sexual fantasy of the allure. In sexual friendships this joining has already taken place. That is, the sexual interaction that one is being allured toward is no longer only the stuff of fantasy, as it is in the allure of strangers and the allure of cross-sex friends. There will obviously still be the fantasy element in the allure of the sexual friend, but it is a fantasy about something that has already taken place. Here the fantasy will be very firmly secured to reality.

When a woman, for example, finds her sexual friend alluring, she will find herself helplessly drawn toward a warm and intimate mixing of her body with his. This bringing together of their bodies will appear to her as a fantasy image that is part of the allure. The image that appears to her, however, need not be one that lies outside her experience. For in his being her sexual friend, she has already had sex with him.

Thus, she has in her memory a collection of numerous images and sequences that lie ready for her fantasy to deploy. Let us say, for example, that the last time they had sex her friend grasped her from behind while kissing her neck and holding her breasts with one hand and her vulva with the other. We could imagine that during this particular sequence she felt herself melt under his caresses, losing the sense of where her body stopped and his began. Because of this, she now has at her disposal a recent and definite image of her sexual interaction with her friend that she finds especially potent. As a consequence, when on a subsequent occasion she notes the allure of her friend, this image will be well situated to reappear suddenly as the fantasy element in the allure she feels. The reasons it is well situated is that, being recent and definite, it is readily available. Were it a distant and vague memory, the chances are that it would be passed over for one with richer features. Also, being an image of an especially arousing embrace—one in which she felt herself melt in his arms—it is naturally the sort of sexual interaction that quickly comes to her mind when she thinks of having sex with her friend again. Further, since this image is of something that actually transpired, it carries with it the sense that it could easily transpire again, especially since the man it took place with is now standing in front of her. This then affects the allure by giving it the sense that the union it is pulling one to will actually materialize.

It should thus be clear that the fantasy element in the allure of a sexual friend is of a different order than the fantasy element in the allure of a stranger. If we think back to the example of my seeing an attractive stranger in the airport lounge, it will be recalled that in finding her sexually attractive, I was instantly brought to the idea of her lips joining with mine, my fingers running through her hair, and so on. These are the sexual fantasies that appear as I fall under the sway of her allure. They are, however, fantasies whose element of interaction has no concrete connection to the woman. For I have never kissed her or run my fingers through her hair. Because of this I have no idea what exactly her specific lips or hair might feel like. I have, however, kissed other women and run my fingers through their hair. Consequently, what my fantasies have done is to take these other concrete experiences and superimpose them onto the stranger I see sitting before me.

This procedure, however, cannot help but give the fantasies a somewhat distant and vague quality, imparting to them a sense of unreality. There are, of course, realistic elements in the fantasy. These are the image of the woman sitting before me and the images of my physical contact with other women. However, in this case the fantasy of allure cannot use these elements unless they are brought together, that is, unless the image of the woman is portrayed as undergoing the physical contact. For the essence of such a fantasy is that it portrays a sexual intermingling of one's own body with that of the sexually attractive person. Yet in this case bringing them together in this way tends to weaken their concreteness and realism. This is simply because of the lack of fit between the two images. It is a lack much like that experienced in watching a dubbed foreign-language film. In such a film the visual images of people talking can be clear and realistic. The same is true of the recording of the voices. However, when the two are brought together, there is always a lack of fit. That is, the mouth movements of the actors do not quite fit with the sounds of the voice recordings. This gives such films an air of unreality, much like the unreality of sexual fantasies involving strangers (which helps to explain why people tend to fantasize about their actual sexual partners).

Things, however, are somewhat different with the fantasies involving cross-sex friends. As I have pointed out, cross-sex friends frequently hug and touch each other, even in sexual ways. This can give someone a concrete image of his own body brought together with the body of his cross-sex friend. This image will clearly help in the formation of a fantasy about sexual contact with his cross-sex friend. However, since the image itself will only be an image of clothed touching, or even sexual touching, it will not, by itself, be an image of having sex. For this to happen, it will have to be embellished with images taken from elsewhere. Thus, here, too, there will be a sense of unreality, though much less so than in that of fantasies about strangers.

Arriving at this point in the discussion, it should now be evident that someone's sexual friendship will have an important effect on the allure that she feels for her friend. In being friends, the attempt to overcome metaphysical isolation is already at work in their relationship. This attempt, which is the basis of the attraction of friendship, works in conjunction with the pull of allure by supporting it. Further, having had sex with her friend before, she will have a good idea of what the sense of being drawn is drawing her to, which will tend to give the pull of allure a sharp and lucid quality. In a similar way, it was shown how the sexual friendship also affected the element of helplessness in allure. Because sexual interaction also contains the element of helplessness, the sense of this helplessness (experienced in the friends' regular sexual interactions) can easily and naturally join with the helplessness felt in allure to give it an intensified prominence. Similarly, since sexual friends have already had sex, the fantasy element of allure will tend to be tied to images of actual sexual encounters with each other. This in turn will tend to affect the allure by giving it a sense of pulling the person toward a goal that will actually be achieved.

This conclusion is echoed by something Vātsyāyana says concerning sexual attraction. He tells us, "Born in both parties at first sight, this attraction grows with the efforts made to realize it." That is, allure, which appears when one first sees the sexually attractive person, does not remain unaffected by one's sexual interactions with the person, but intensifies with efforts to realize the goal of the allure, namely, sexual union. "This kind of attraction," he says, "is also found on returning from a journey, or on meeting again after a quarrel."[34] These are good examples because on returning from a journey, one is returning to something, say one's sexual partner, whom one knows previously by direct acquaintance. The same is true for meeting after a quarrel. After the quarrel one had been distant from one's partner, but in meeting again, one has joined with her once more. In the same way, the allure of one's sexual friend is a returning to or meeting again (through the pull of allure) something (an intimate joining of bodies) that one knows from previous experience.

FIVE

It Turned Out So Right

ROMANTIC ATTRACTION

Throughout this study I have several times referred to romantic love. This was something that came naturally in the course of discussions about sexual attraction even though they might not have been discussions about romantic love itself. The reason is the particularly close connections that romantic love and sexual attraction enjoy, which I have already noted in the first chapter. Because of these connections, it is difficult to discuss sexual attraction without making reference to romantic love. But how is it that romantic love and sexual attraction have come to have such close ties? To be able to answer this question, we must first have an idea of what constitutes romantic love.

One thing that is obviously involved in romantic love is something I have referred to several times, namely, romantic attraction. It is, however, difficult to see exactly how these two things are related. This is because the terms "romantic love" and "romantic attraction" are not used in clearly distinct ways. In one way, "romantic love" is often used to refer to the entire psychological and physical phenomenon that takes place when one person is in love with another. "Romantic attraction" can also be used this way. But on the other hand, it seems it is often used to refer to just the phenomenon of being attracted to the person with whom one is in love, rather than to the entire relationship.

Romantic attraction also differs from love in another way. For it seems one can be romantically attracted to someone whom one is not fully in love with but only attracted to as a possible romantic partner, as, for example, when one person is courting another. There is the typical example of the man who is besotted with a particular woman and attempts to show her his romantic intentions by texting her, sending her cards, buying her gifts, and trying to arrange meetings with her. Depending, however, on the intensity of his desires, it might not be correct to say he is romantically in love. Rather, even though he is enamored with her, he could be simply showing his interest while waiting to see how she feels about him, even trying to encourage romantic desires in her, before he lets himself fall fully in love with her. In this sort of case, even though it might not be correct to say he is in love with her, it does seem correct to say he is romantically attracted to her. Romantic attraction therefore has a wider application than does romantic love. However, even in those cases where romantic attraction is not experienced within an established love relationship, it is nevertheless fundamentally connected to love. This is because in being romantically attracted to another person, one is attracted to the other person as a possible or actual romantic partner—in other words, as a possible or actual romantic lover.

It is important to see, however, that not all instances of courting or showing apparent romantic attraction are necessarily instances of real romantic attraction. People can seek out ostensible romantic partners for reasons that have nothing to do with romantic attraction. A single woman in her late 20s, for example, might suddenly be aware that all her friends are now married. Perhaps she has even just finished being a bridesmaid for the third time, thus becoming all too aware of the saying "Three times a bridesmaid, never a bride." This could also involve anxieties about wanting to be a mother while feeling that time is running out. In such a case, she might then start desperately looking about to see who is still available and, vaguely remembering a man who showed her some interest a few years ago (but to whom she felt no attraction), seek him out and try to revive his interest.

Her seeking him out, however, has nothing to do with romantic attraction, though she will naturally try to convince the man, others, and maybe even herself that she is romantically attracted to him. Rather, her behavior is driven by her fear of ending up single and appearing to be a woman no man wanted. It is worth noting that in Japanese culture the same concern is expressed in the saying "Nobody wants leftover Christmas cake," that is, nobody will purchase Christmas cake after 25 December. This is used to warn a girl that if she wants a partner, she had better find one before she is 25 years old, because after 25 no one will want her. She would then be in the same position as leftover Christmas cake. One could imagine that as her 25th birthday approaches, a single Japanese girl might let romantic attraction fall to the wayside as she rushes about trying to find a partner.

Or again, there might be a man who appears to show romantic attraction to a woman, doing what he can to get her to fall in love with him, and yet really has no romantic attraction to her at all. In such a case it might be that his friends think she is "hot," even though he himself does not find her attractive. Consequently, he is aware that if he were to acquire her as a girlfriend, his status among his friends would be much increased. Again, as in the example of the woman just mentioned, he might even try to deceive himself into believing he is actually in love with her.

It could also be the case, for both men and women, that someone is unsuccessful in getting the particular individual he or she is romantically attracted to. As a result, rather than remain single, the person might settle for someone he or she can get, even though that person is not seen to be romantically attractive. Something like this is the idea behind the "level of aspiration" explanation for the matching hypothesis that was discussed in the first chapter. This is the idea that people tend to choose partners who are at their own level of attractiveness because of their resignation to the fact that they cannot attract persons of a higher level of attractiveness.

It could even happen that someone decides on choosing a partner he finds unattractive. Perhaps, for example, he has been through a string of unhappy romances with sexually attractive women, romances in which each of the women has left him or been taken from him by another man. He might then come to the idea that sexually attractive women are just too much bother and too difficult to keep. Rather than pursue yet another attractive woman and risk losing her, he might choose a sexually unattractive woman. For, his reasoning might go, not only is such a woman easy to win, but there is little risk in her leaving him for another man or in another man wanting her.

In cases like these, romantic attraction plays little or no role in the formation of a couple, even though both others and the couple themselves will probably refer to themselves as lovers, boyfriend and girlfriend, or romantic partners.

An example of the pragmatic basis behind seemingly romantic choices is nicely captured in a song by Jimi Hendrix in which he describes coming home to find out his "baby" has left him. He is not, however, too bothered, not only because he still has his guitar, but also because, as he explains in the closing line of the song, "If my baby don't love me no more, I know her sister will!"

Because of all this, it is important to remember that not all apparently romantic relationships are set in motion by romantic attraction. This is important because if we want to understand the nature of romantic attraction, it is vital that we do not get led astray by attempting to accommodate these other sorts of relationships in an account of romantic attraction but keep focused on actual instances of romantic attraction. A similar problem was encountered in the first chapter with regard to sexual attraction. There I showed how certain cases of apparent sexual attraction were really attraction to other things such as possessions, wealth, or status.

But if romantic attraction is the process of being attracted to the person with whom one is in love or at least wants to be in love, and if sexual attraction is part of romantic attraction, what then is the distinction between romantic attraction and sexual attraction? That there is such a distinction should be obvious from the discussion so far. Yet throughout the literature, scholars often fail to make this distinction. Many studies, for example, claim to be investigating romantic attraction when it is unclear whether they are examining romantic attraction or sexual attraction. Sometimes they are just investigating sexual attraction even though they call it romantic attraction. The reason for not clearly drawing this distinction is probably that, as I argued in the first pages of this book, sexual attraction is an integral part of romantic attraction. This means that when someone is romantically attracted to another person, he or she is at the same time sexually attracted to that person. Consequently, when a scholar is discussing romantic attraction, much of what is being said also applies to sexual attraction. This makes it easy enough to overlook the distinction between the two.

A difficulty appears, however, because although sexual attraction is part of romantic attraction, romantic attraction is not part of sexual attraction. That is, someone can easily feel sexual attraction to another person without being romantically attracted to him or her. This is obvious from what has been shown in the previous chapters, namely that one can have sexual attraction to strangers, cross-sex friends, and sexual friends, none of whom one need be attracted to as a romantic partner. One can, of course, come to develop romantic feelings for any such individuals, even instantly, as love at first sight shows. But again, such a development need not happen. However, it is important to note that sexually attractive strangers, cross-sex friends, and sexual friends all hold a privileged position as potential romantic partners. This is because they already have the fundamental quality required for romantic attraction, namely, being sexually attractive. And, as Aristotle reminds us, "no one loves if he has not first been delighted by the form of the beloved."

But if romantic attraction is more than just sexual attraction, what more is it? One expected reply here is that in addition to sexual attraction to the person's physical appearance, it is attraction to the personality or personality traits. In this view what one is romantically attracted to in another person is, in addition to the person's physical appearance (which is the sexual part of romantic attraction), things like the person's kindness, warmth, sense of humor, and so on. Such a view might seem supported by the fact that people often say things about their romantic partners such as, "What attracted me to Sarah was her generosity, helpfulness, and openness to new ideas," all of which refer to personality traits.

The difficulty with this, however, is that the same thing is true for friendship. That is, what people are attracted to in their friends is also their personality traits. But if this is the case, how are we to distinguish between romantic attraction and the attraction of friendship? It will not help to point to the sexual activity that often takes place, or even the sexual attraction that exists in romantic attraction, because as we have seen, this also takes place in cross-sex friendships and sexual friendships.

One way to make this distinction, it might seem, would be to see romantic attraction as a more intense version of the same attraction one feels in friendship. Therefore, to be romantically attracted to someone is just the same as liking a friend, with the exception that the romantic attraction is a more intense liking. There are, however, several points that count against such an easy distinction.

For one thing, friendship does not seem to be dependent on gender in the way that romantic attraction is. Most people can easily have friends of both genders, but most people are not romantically attracted to persons of both genders. That is, gender seems to play a crucial role in romantic attraction, but not in friendship.

Also, romantic attraction seems to involve a continuous fantasizing about being together with the romantic partner, imagining what it would be like to be in her presence, to see her smile, to look into her eyes, and so on. Friendship seldom involves this sort of fantasizing about future meetings and going over them in detail. Of course, in cross-sex friendships or especially sexual friendships, there will be fantasizing about the sexual aspects of the relationship, but not, it seems, about just being with the person and the details of future encounters. A cross-sex or sexual friendship might well come to this, but then it would appear to have crossed over into a romantic relationship.

Further, there is both a volatility and a swiftness of onset and decline in romantic attraction that tends to be absent in friendships. Friendships, both same-sex and cross-sex, tend to have a stability that is less common in romantic relationships. People are forever falling in love, having affairs, and breaking up, while friendships are not so volatile. Friends can fall out with each other, but this is far less common than the termination of love affairs. Also, friendships tend to form and terminate gradually in a way that is not true of romantic attraction.

In addition, although negative experiences surrounding a friend or a friendship will tend to lead to an abandonment of the friendship, such experiences can have the opposite effect in romantic attraction. Here, the lack of interest in or even abusive behavior toward one partner by the other can lead the person to grasp more desperately at the uninterested partner with intensified feelings of love. This is the dynamic referred to earlier in the song lyrics "You treat me badly, I love you madly." This sort of intensification of romantic feelings seems based on a fear of losing the lover. For as the neglect or mistreatment sets in, the person becomes aware that a possible termination of the relationship lays just beyond the horizon. Being still in love and thus not wanting to lose the other person, his or her romantic feelings reassert themselves with all their strength. I have discussed these points in terms of romantic love more fully elsewhere, and so will not go deeper into them here.[1]

Finally, as we have seen, one does not need to like or to be friends with one's lover. This alone seems to be enough to show that romantic attraction cannot simply be an intense form of liking. For in such cases we have romantic attraction with no liking.

What, then, remains of romantic attraction when it is considered apart from the sexual attraction it involves? The answer, I should like to suggest, is that what remains is the psychological counterpart to sexual attraction. In other words, what remains is attraction to a psychological version of what one is attracted to in sexual attraction. This, however, is only a theoretical consideration. For in reality, the psychological aspect of romantic love, as I shall argue shortly, never appears without the sexual aspect faithfully at its side or, to be more correct, faithfully in its midst. In sexual attraction what one is attracted to is the idea of the other person's body brought together with one's own body. This conjoining of bodies is seen to be accomplished through a mutual baring and caressing, which are themselves the physical expression of vulnerability and care. For in baring my body to my sexual partner, I am vulnerable before her, as is she before me when she bares her body to me. And in caressing each other's nakedness, we simultaneously show care to each other.

The psychological counterpart of this is when we open ourselves psychologically and emotionally to each other. This is typically done by romantic partners through participating in things like intimate exchanges, trust, and sharing of personal feelings. For in becoming intimate and close with someone, putting oneself in his or her trust, and sharing private feelings with him or her, one has become psychologically and emotionally vulnerable to him or her. And just as one becomes naked before one's sexual partner in order to be caressed, so one becomes psychologically vulnerable before one's romantic partner in order that she may be supportive, listen, offer help, and show concern—in other words, in order that she may care. Further, and this is the crucial part, not only does one become vulnerable in this way, but one *desires* to become vulnerable. Why? So that one's romantic partner can show the desired care. In just the same way, one desires one's partner to desire to become psychologically vulnerable before oneself in order that one can show care to her. That is, one has desires concerning the other person's desires. One desires that the beloved has the same desires toward oneself that one has toward her. This is the reciprocity inherent in romantic love. When such desires are not reciprocated, there appears the well-known pain of unrequited love.

I should also point out here that although I refer to the act of opening oneself emotionally to one's beloved, this does not imply that love itself is an emotion. I say this because although love is often seen as an emotion, many people do not experience love in an emotional way. Various emotions can attend the experience of love, and this would seem especially so for someone who is emotionally disposed. But the feelings that usually go with love—for example, elation, euphoria, and butterflies in the stomach—are peripheral to the essence of love.

It is this complex of reciprocal desires involving the romantically attractive person that makes up the other (nonsexual) half of romantic attraction. It is the psychological counterpart to the sexual attraction one lover feels for the other. A person in love is therefore romantically attracted not only to an intimate exchange of physical vulnerability and care (baring and caressing) with the beloved but also, as a further expression of this, to an intimate exchange of psychological vulnerability and care. Furthermore, just as sexual attraction can be of varying degrees, so can romantic attraction also be of varying degrees (since it is based on sexual attraction). Although we tend to think of romantic attraction in terms of its more powerful expressions, romantic attraction can well assume different degrees, depending on various factors. The strength of the attraction will depend on things such as the circumstances or the personality of the individual undergoing the experience.

None of this is to say that vulnerability and care are the only things that figure in the experience of romantic attraction. Of course, there are qualities about an individual's personality that one finds attractive in a romantic partner—perhaps her generosity, helpfulness, and openness to new ideas.

But these are only romantically attractive so far as they are traits of a person who also attracts one to engage in an exchange of mutual psychological vulnerability and care. And one is only attracted to this exchange if one is first sexually attracted to the person. Ignoring the sexual element in romantic attraction, this attraction to such an exchange would be the core difference between the attraction of friendship and romantic attraction. For in friendship one is attracted to the particular personality traits of one's friend, not in order to exchange mutual vulnerability and care with one's friend, but simply because those personality traits are what one enjoys about one's friend. Friends can, of course, on various occasions be vulnerable before each other, but this is neither something they desire nor something that is the basis of their attraction to each other (or if it is, then one should question whether it is just a friendship). In romantic attraction, however, one is attracted precisely to an exchange of mutual vulnerability and care with a particular person (who will display particular personality traits one enjoys).

This should not be taken to mean that there are no gray areas between friendship and love. As we have seen, cross-sex friendships and sexual friendships are quite capable of going on to become romantic relationships. And although romantic love tends to be swift in its onset, there can still be periods where it is unclear to someone in such a friendship whether what she is experiencing is still just the liking of friendship. For maybe she might wonder if murmurings of romantic attraction are beginning to make themselves heard. In such a situation she might well be in a friendship that is, as the title of one film put it, a lot like love. Things even become more complex when it is remembered that romantic partners can also be friends. This is something I will come to shortly. But although romantic attraction and the attraction of friendship are distinct, romantic attraction and sexual attraction are not. It is true that romantic attraction is more than sexual attraction, but, as I argued in the first chapter, sexual attraction is still an integral part of romantic attraction.

From what has been said so far, it should be clear that sexual attraction and the nonsexual aspect of romantic attraction share a similar structure. Sexual attraction is the attraction to mutual vulnerability and care in the form of mutual baring and caressing. This is the physical expression of mutual vulnerability and care. The nonsexual aspect of romantic attraction, on the other hand, is the attraction to mutual vulnerability and care in the form of mutual psychological intimacy and showing of concern. This is the psychological expression of mutual vulnerability and care. The reason why sexual attraction is an integral part of romantic attraction is that sexual attraction is the basis from which love grows. Consequently, if there is romantic attraction, then there must also be sexual attraction.

One could always raise the question, however, of why the nonsexual aspect of romantic attraction could not exist on its own without the sexual aspect. Or to put it another way, why cannot someone experience romantic attraction toward someone without experiencing the sexual attraction toward her? The answer is that romantic attraction gets its force from sexual attraction. That is, the romantic attraction I feel toward someone is driven by the sexual attraction I feel toward her. The relationship between romantic attraction and sexual attraction is much like the relationship between the root of a plant and the plant's foliage. As long as the root is connected to the foliage, the foliage with continue to grow. However, were the foliage to be cut off from the root, losing its base from which to grow, the foliage would quickly shrivel and die. In the same way, as long as there is sexual attraction, romantic attraction receives its nourishment and continues to live, but without sexual attraction, romantic attraction will quickly shrivel and die.

Of course, someone could question this and ask why romantic attraction cannot generate its own nourishment. Why does it need sexual attraction to stay alive? And here the answer would seem to be that one needs the concrete and definite object of sexual attraction in order to give love it's forceful and focused direction. The idea of two naked bodies intimately joined immediately and easily wrests our attention away from other concerns in a way that two minds in psychological intimacy do not. This is because the image or fantasy of oneself in an intimate embrace with a sexually attractive person is something we have no problem conjuring up. Indeed, it seems to appear spontaneously and of its own accord. However, the image of oneself in a state of psychological intimacy and concern with a romantically attractive person seems less precise and difficult to picture. There does not appear to be a definite event here that comes to mind as a goal. Perhaps an exchange of romantic desires or associated emotions might be something we imagine, but such notions by themselves lack the definiteness to become the image of the goal in the experience of romantic attraction. Or at least they lack such definiteness when compared to the image of two naked bodies in a sexual embrace.

Because of this lack of definiteness, and also because of the similarity between romantic and sexual attraction, it seems romantic attraction naturally focuses on the object of sexual attraction instead of an image of nonsexual romantic interaction. Thus, when I ask people to give an account of what they are attracted to when they feel romantic attraction, the answer typically involves something like embracing, kissing, or being physically intimate with the beloved. But these are just the images and fantasies used in sexual attraction. The difference is that in nonromantic sexual attraction (say, to strangers or cross-sex friends), these fantasies are typically not attended by desires concerning mutual psychological vulnerability and care, while in romantic attraction they are. Nevertheless, the images of sexual attraction are already embedded in the images of romantic attraction. In this way the force of the sexual aspect of romantic attraction is easily transferred to the nonsexual aspect. Consequently, to feel romantic attraction is at the same time to feel sexual attraction. This is why someone cannot be romantically attracted to another without also being sexually attracted to him or her.

Further support for this view comes from a simple examination of the individual to whom one is romantically attracted. This is because the individual to whom one is romantically attracted is always specific (though one, of course, can be romantically attracted to more than one specific individual). And specific individuals tend to have specific genders. (This is also true for transgendered and intersexed persons, for they, too, have specific genders, namely, transgender and intersex.) Consequently, what one is romantically attracted to is someone of a specific gender. Further, it is crucial for most people that the person of their romantic affections is of a specific gender. Therefore, a heterosexual, for example, will tend to find it exceedingly important that the person that he or she falls in love with will be of the opposite sex. But why should this be such an issue? Why should it matter if the person with whom one has an exchange of mutual psychological vulnerability and care is one sex rather than another? The answer is that the attraction to an exchange of mutual psychological vulnerability does not occur independently of the attraction to an exchange of mutual physical vulnerability and care. Or in other words, the psychological aspect of romantic attraction does not take place without the sexual aspect. That is, the reason the sex of one's romantic partner is important is that the sex of one's sexual partner is important. And one's romantic partner *is* one's (actual or potential) sexual partner.

With this it also becomes clear why romantic partners need not be friends, for a central part of any friendship is mutual liking. And mutual liking consists of, among other things, companionship or the enjoyment of each other's company for its own sake. But there is nothing in an exchange of mutual psychological vulnerability and care between two people that implies such an enjoyment of each other's company. One can be attracted to or desire another person's vulnerability in order to show care and yet have no obvious enjoyment of the person's company simply for the sake of being with him.

One just wants the other person to be in a state where she needs one's care. And the same is true of the other desires of wanting oneself to be vulnerable in order to be cared for and desiring that the other person reciprocate with similar desires toward oneself. Typically, there is an enjoyment in the exchange of mutual vulnerability and care, but there need not be. There might even be an unpleasantness attending the exchange. Such a dimension would seem to manifest itself in those instances where one of romantic partners fears the loss of the other, which in turn leads to an intensification of his or her romantic desires. Here the attraction can take on an anxious and desperate quality. It might well be these sorts of instances that are referred to by the well-known expression "Love hurts." It is because of cases like these that romantic attraction cannot be defined in terms of enjoyment.

Moreover, the seeking of each other's company in romantic attraction is not even clearly an instance of seeking companionship, at least in the sense of wanting to be with someone simply for the sake of being with her. For in romantic attraction the lover is attracted to the beloved for the fundamental purpose of an exchange of mutual vulnerability and care (that is, to share romantic love), not for friendship.

An excellent example of this is found in what is probably the most famous love story of all, Shakespeare's play *Romeo and Juliet*.[2] For although Romeo and Juliet are clearly deeply in love, they are just as clearly not friends. And here it is important to remember that their not being friends does not mean that they are enemies. It simply means that friendship is not part of their relationship to each other. To see this, consider how their relationship develops. Romeo first sees Juliet from a distance while at a party. Entranced with her beauty, he instantly falls in love with her. He then approaches her, and they get to talk, touch, and kiss briefly. Juliet then quickly falls in love with Romeo. When later leaving the building, Romeo is thrilled to see Juliet at a window, and they exchange vows. They then meet for a secret wedding in a friar's cell and quickly part company. Later that evening Romeo sneaks into Juliet's bedroom, and they spend their wedding night together, during which they have sex. That is the last time they interact. In an effort to help them be together, the friar concocts a plan that will make Juliet appear to be dead so that she can later run away with Romeo. Romeo, however, does not know of the plan and believes Juliet is actually dead. Coming upon her apparently lifeless body (which is merely anesthetized with a sleeping potion), Romeo falls into despair and commits suicide. Upon awakening from her drug-induced sleep, Juliet discovers Romeo's actually lifeless body and, in a moment of desperation, takes her own life.

It is fascinating to note that, in all this flurry of desire and craving for each other, there is no inkling of friendship. Juliet does refer to Romeo at one point as "love, lord, ay, husband, friend" (just before he is to slip away after having spent the night), but the word "friend" is used rather loosely throughout the play, and there is little to suggest they have any relation of friendship over and above their romantic and sexual relationship. Clearly, they wish each other well and are inclined, so far as they can, to bring these things about. But what is lacking is companionship, that is, an enjoyment of each other's company for its own sake. Of course, they enjoy each other's company. But this is enjoyed because it enables them to fulfill their romantic desires, that is, desires for an exchange of mutual vulnerability and care. Companionship, however, involves the enjoyment of being together simply for the sake of each other's company. They do not show any sense of this sort of enjoyment and therefore no sense of companionship.

It is also unclear how much they show other commonly cited elements of friendship, such as safety, support, understanding, and shared activities. And in a way, this is understandable because they only meet four times, briefly and secretly at that, with minimal chance for openness, self-disclosure, and sharing of personal information. Although this is no hindrance to the onset of romantic love, it is a hindrance to the development of friendship. For unlike romantic love, friendship tends to be gradual in its appearance. Friendships tend to form slowly as the friends engage in discussions, openness, reciprocal self-disclosure, and participation in shared activities. In the star-crossed lovers' whirlwind romance, there is simply no time or opportunity for such things to take place, especially when what opportunities they do have are used rather to explore and express their love for one another and have sex. This shows clearly, then, that friendship need not be part of romantic love and thus that people can be deeply in love with one another without being friends.

It might be thought, however, that, if the friar's plan had not been botched, and Romeo and Juliet had managed to run off and live out their days together, they would have eventually become friends. For somehow, it might be thought, the desires of love would have eventually influenced the development of friendship. Yet nothing in their romantic relationship implies that a development of friendship need take place. Romeo and Juliet could simply go on being romantically in love, exchanging mutual vulnerability and care, without ever developing the mutual liking that is the hallmark of friends. Of course, the intensity of their romantic attraction may dissipate over time, settling into a less passionate version of romantic love. But, again, this need not bring friendship along with it.

Therefore, were someone to meet Romeo years later (assuming the friar's plan had worked) and suggest that by now he had certainly become friends with his deeply loved wife, Romeo could still happily reply (in harmony with the subject cited earlier), "I don't think that friendship has anything to do with marriage [or love]. I wouldn't want my wife to be my best friend. I think as a wife she should respect me and treat me the way a good wife should."

Someone might feel, of course, that this assertion is antiromantic. It sounds cold and distant, with the ideas of "respect" and expectations about the way "a good wife" should treat her husband, making it look like he sees his wife as more of a servant than a romantic partner. Accordingly, it might be concluded that not only would a man with such a view lack friendship with his wife but, further, he could not be in love with her.

This, however, need not be the case. For as far as romantic love goes, holding such a view is quite compatible with desires for mutual vulnerability and care. In this case, what the person desires is reciprocity in terms of an exchange of vulnerability and care, not necessarily reciprocity in other areas. In the same way, it is quite possible for someone to be in love with his servant (especially if the other person is happy to take the role of a servant). Still, the fact that someone in such a relationship is in love should not be taken to imply that the relationship will thereby be a happy one. To be sure, people in these sorts of loving but friendless of relationships will most likely not be happy. This is the truth seen by the German philosopher Friedrich Nietzsche, who says, "It is not a lack of love, but a lack of friendship that makes unhappy marriages."[3]

One of the difficulties in accepting the idea that romantic lovers need not become friends is that some people have referred to a less passionate version of romantic love as companionate love. This is a version of romantic love that can gradually appear over the course of a romantic relationship. This might make it sound like romantic lovers naturally become companions, and therefore friends, as time goes by. However, the word "companionate" is not here being used in the way that I am using the word "companionship," something that I have argued refers to a core feature of friendship. Social psychologists Elaine Hatfield and G. William Walster, for example, define companionate love as "the affection we feel for those with whom our lives are deeply entwined."[4] Plainly, there is nothing in this definition that necessarily implies friendship. The affection mentioned here could simply be a less intensified version of the complex of romantic desires that I have been referring to. Also, having one's life deeply entwined with another sounds slightly more like the interactions of romantic love (or perhaps family relations) than those of friendship.

At the same time, however, none of this shows that romantic love and friendship cannot occur together. In many cases of romantic love there is a clear enjoyment of each other's companionship, with the romantic partners even being best friends. Here the friendship may develop more or less hand in hand with the romance (though the romantic relationship will tend to have a swifter onset). In many cases, as we have seen with both cross-sex and sexual friendships, friends go on to be romantic partners, which need not mean the friendship disappears but only that a romantic relationship is added to it. Or again, the friendship may only come after the romantic love is already firmly established. Thus, if the friar's plan had not been bungled, and Romeo and Juliet had managed to run off and live out their days together, they might well have eventually become friends. They might have developed a sense of companionship, engaged in openness, reciprocal self-disclosure, and participated in shared activities. If they had kept their love alive while this gestation of friendship took place, then they could have become both lovers and friends.

Despite its being obvious that friendship and love occur together in these various ways, there are some who nevertheless think that romantic love and friendship are incompatible. An example of this view is given by the philosopher James Conlon in an article entitled "Why lovers can't be friends." Here Conlon rejects the idea that one's lover can also be one's friend. His reason for this is that the two relationships are mutually exclusive. To explain why he thinks this, he uses an analogy with literary genres. Human relationships, he says, are much like different types of literature. For just as there are distinct genres of literature (poems, plays, novels, and so on), so are there distinct sorts of relationships (work relationships, friendship, love, and so on). Novels and poems, he argues, are distinct and incommensurable genres, and it is the genre's limits that give it its meaning. The value of a poem would be lost, he tells us, if it tried to be a novel. He then applies this idea to human relationships, claiming that love and friendship are distinct genres of intimacy: "Like the poem and the novel, they cannot be combined." In explaining why they cannot be combined he asserts that "friends share each other's experience of the world; they see it in similar ways and enjoy it together." But "In love, one does not so much delight in sharing separate experiences, as want every experience, even the most minute, not to be separate."[5]

This argument, however, is quite unconvincing. In the first place, it is not true that poems and novels cannot be combined. *Alice's Adventures in Wonderland* is a novel that has poems combined with it. Further, the poems are integral parts of the novel, using their fantasy, nonsense, and neologisms to transport the reader into the marvelous world of a seven-year-old. But perhaps Conlon does not mean that a poem cannot be embedded within a novel, but rather that a single poem cannot itself be the same thing as a novel. But if this is what he means, then here, too, he would be wrong. Epic poems are very close to the idea of a poem that is also a novel. *The Odyssey*, for example, has main characters and a storyline, begins in medias res, and has flashbacks and nonlinear narratives, all of which are devices typically used in novels. Yet *The Odyssey* also has the metric lines typical of classical poetry. As a consequence, if love is like a poem and friendship like a novel, then the analogy would suggest that love and friendship can indeed be combined.

I also do not see why lovers cannot delight in sharing experiences the way friends do. Like friends, lovers can also see the world in similar ways and enjoy it together. Of course, lovers also want to feel unified with each other, seeing the world through each other's eyes, as it were. But this is only incompatible with the sharing of each other's experiences if one attempts to do both at the same time. Yet there is no reason why a person need attempt this. In one moment when I feel particularly close to my lover, I might well long to experience the moment as she does. But in other situations I might want to hear about how she undergoes the moment from her own point of view, to find out about her (and enjoy her way of seeing things), rather than seek to identify with it.

That the desire to unify with the beloved does not need to fill every situation is supported by the existence of polyamory, or the state of being romantically in love with more than one person at one time. Although many people tend to think of romantic love as being an exclusive experience in which a person can experience romantic love for only one person at a time, it need not be. People can easily be in love with more than one person at once. Western cultural norms are against these sorts of relationships, often forcing a person to think she cannot really love more than one person and therefore must choose. But this is a requirement of Western cultural norms, not of romantic love. Because of this possibility of being in love with more than one person, it seems wrong to say that romantic love necessarily involves the desire to always experience the world as the lover does. For if one has two or three persons with whom one is in love, then one should want always to experience the world in two or three separate ways at the same time. But this does not make sense. So, it is unclear in this view what the person in love is supposed to be wanting.

LOVERS AND FRIENDS

With this it should now be plain that lovers can easily be friends. Not only does one hear people continually referring to their lover or spouse as their good or even best friend, but common elements of friendship, such as support, loyalty, constancy, understanding, and shared activities, seem to lend themselves naturally to the love relationship. This suggests that there is some basic connection between friendship and romantic attraction. Yet, as I have shown, romantic partners need not be friends. This would indicate that there is no fundamental connection. But what, then, is the relationship between friendship and romantic attraction?

To answer this question, we can start by recalling that the origin of friendship is the deep sense of metaphysical isolation that each of us has. This leads us to come as close as possible to another awareness by seeking out the mutual liking of friendship. The origin of romantic attraction, however, is quite different. Here, the primary component is that of sexual attraction. This attraction, which is the attraction to an exchange of bodily vulnerability and care (that is, baring and caressing), spills over into the attraction to an exchange of psychological vulnerability and care (that is, psychological intimacy and concern. I will come to why this occurs in the next section). This differs from the roots of friendship in two important ways.

First, there is no sexual attraction component to friendship. Sexual attraction can go together with friendship, but it is not the essence of friendship in the way that it is the essence of romantic attraction. Secondly, while friendship is based on the attempt to overcome metaphysical isolation, this plays no part in the essence of romantic attraction. Of course, romantic attraction also looks like an attempt to overcome metaphysical isolation, for it, too, is an attempt to get as close to another person as possible. Whether or not lovers are friends, they still want to spend time together and to develop a closeness and intimacy with each other.

However, the closeness and intimacy aimed at in romantic attraction is of a different order than that of friendship. With romantic attraction it is an attempt to get as close as possible to a person of a particular gender; with heterosexuals it is the opposite gender while with homosexuals it is the same gender. In both cases it is the element of gender that plays the decisive role. The goal here is to achieve a closeness and intimacy with someone who is a male or someone who is a female. In other words, romantic attraction is not so much an attempt to overcome metaphysical isolation as it is a movement toward overcoming gender isolation. This is why it is crucial for people (including bisexuals, as follows from the evidence surrounding bisexuals and sexual attraction) that the person they fall in love with is of a particular gender. What catches someone's eye first about a possible romantic partner is the person's gender. In the instant this is determined, or rather a microsecond later, the person's sexual attractiveness is decided upon (though this might be reevaluated with subsequent information). Only when this has taken place can the person be seen as a possible romantic partner. This process of noting gender, sexual attractiveness, and then romantic attractiveness may evidently take place one after the other, or instantaneously, as in the case of love at first sight (though even here my guess would be that our cognitive processing notes gender first before rapidly noting sexual attractiveness and then immediately proceeding to romantic attractiveness).

This sequence is dramatically displayed in *Romeo and Juliet* when Romeo first spots the girl of his dreams. The primacy of the element of gender in the sequence is shown when, upon seeing her, he asks a servant, "What lady is that . . . ?," thus indicating his noting of her gender. He then immediately says, "O, she doth teach the torches to burn bright!" referring to her sexual attractiveness. And, since the object of sexual attraction is one's own body brought together with the attractive person's body, he immediately fantasizes the joining of their bodies, saying, "And, touching hers, make blessed my rude hand." In the next instant his romantic attraction appears as he proclaims, "Did my heart love till now? forswear it, sight!" And just to remind us that romantic love flows from sexual attraction, he explains his declaration of love by saying, "For I ne'er saw true beauty till this night."

Just as one could challenge the idea that gender plays a decisive role in sexual attraction, so can one challenge the idea that gender plays a decisive role in romantic attraction. Someone could claim, for example, that there are people who are romantically attracted to others regardless of their gender. Perhaps, the person might continue, such individuals are romantically attracted to other nongender aspects of the person. Although there might be people who believe this about themselves, I feel that a careful examination of the romantic attraction in such instances would reveal that gender is still a determining factor. In the film *The Crying Game*, to take a well-known example, the story involves a man, Fergus, who develops a romantic attraction to Dil, someone who Fergus thinks is a woman. And at one point Dil, without taking off her clothes, performs oral sex on Fergus. Later, however, during another sexual encounter, Fergus discovers that Dil has a penis and is in fact a man. He responds to this with shock and disgust and even vomits before leaving. Eventually, however, he becomes aware that he still is romantically attracted to Dil and returns to him. Interestingly, however, they do not end up together because in "taking the rap" for a shooting done by Dil, Fergus ends up in jail.

In this story it is easy to think that what Fergus is romantically attracted to is Dil as a person, regardless of his gender. This, it might be thought, is why his romantic attraction to Dil is able to persist even after he discovers that Dil is not a woman but is in fact just a man dressed as a woman. I feel, however, there are better explanations. One explanation is based on the idea that Fergus is bisexual. This would seem to be the case, since he is apparently able to be romantically attracted to both women and men. I say this because it could be thought, on the contrary, that he is simply a heterosexual who is attracted to persons regardless of their gender. But if he is attracted to persons regardless of their gender, what is the point of calling him heterosexual? For the definitive point about being heterosexual is that one is sexually and romantically attracted to the opposite sex. It might be that he originally believed he was heterosexual, but upon encountering Dil discovered that he was more or less bisexual, or even turned bisexual. But even so, the point remains that in dealing with Dil as a man, he is now romantically attracted to him as a man. In both instances, when he first thinks Dil is a woman and when he later discovers he is a man, the basis of his romantic attraction to Dil is Dil's apparent gender. This view, I think, is even supported by the fact that immediately upon discovering Dil's male genitals during a sexual interaction, Fergus becomes disgusted and vomits. If he was romantically attracted to Dil regardless of Dil's gender, why would he be disgusted? If what he was attracted to had little to do with Dil's gender, then plainly he would just take this in his stride and merely adjust his sexual activity to accommodate his partner's male genitals and lack of a vagina.

Now, of course, there will be bisexuals who can do this, but even here it would seem that, according to the research, bisexuals still have to put themselves in a different mindset in order to focus on "the something unique or different" that each gender has to offer. That Fergus responds to Dil's maleness by vomiting suggests both that he has not shifted from his heterosexual gear and that at this point he is probably not aware of his own bisexuality. Later, coming to terms with this discovery about himself, he is then able to "shift gears" and make a romantic return to Dil.

Another possible interpretation is that rather than being bisexual, Fergus is homosexual but, at the beginning of the film, is unaware of or has repressed his own homosexuality. For it is common enough that people, even in our own supposedly enlightened times, still hide their homosexuality not only from others but also from themselves. Later, then, with the help of his encounter with Dil, he is able to become aware of and accept his homosexuality. If Fergus were an actual person, then just which of these interpretations is correct could only be decided through discussions with him and engaging him in a psychological analysis. For my purposes, the important thing is that both of these interpretations fit with what we know from the research. Such events as these therefore do not force us to accept the unsupported view that people are romantically attracted to others regardless of their gender.

The plausible conclusion to draw from all this is that it is the attempt to overcome gender isolation that is the driving force behind romantic attraction. The attempt to overcome gender isolation provides this force, as I argued a few pages ago, by being the basis of the sexual attraction that is itself the basis of romantic attraction.

But having established this does not help with the main problem of understanding how friendship and romantic attraction seem to go so well together. It merely allows us to draw a negative conclusion, namely that whatever makes romantic attraction and friendship go together, it cannot be that they both are a reaction to the same sense of metaphysical isolation. In fact, it seems to even put us further away from achieving this understanding by assuring us that romantic attraction and friendship spring from very different sources, namely, an awareness of metaphysical isolation and an awareness of gender isolation.

All, however, is not lost. For the answer lies, I think, in noting that romantic partners and friends share an important feature in common. This is the simple feature of spending time together. For one of the things about spending time together is that it encourages liking. The question of whether spending time together leads mainly to liking or disliking is one that is often discussed (much like the question of whether men and women can be just friends). Here arguments are given to show how the more you see someone, the more he or she "rubs off on you" or, taking the contrary position, how "familiarity breeds contempt."

The problem with such discussions is that there are often numerous examples that seem to support each position. When, however, we turn to the available research, it seems that the familiarity that results from spending time together mainly leads to liking. Several studies have shown that merely increasing someone's exposure to another person results in his or her developing a liking for that person. One classic study, for example, demonstrated that people were twice as likely to become friends with someone who lived within 20 feet of them than they were with people who lived within 40 feet of them.[6] The obvious explanation for this is that such proximity enabled them to see each other more. The increase in exposure alone was enough to lead to an increase in liking. Although some studies have shown that proximity can also be related to disliking, in such cases it seems to be factors like "environmental spoiling," where one person disturbs another person's arrangements or activities, that are to blame.[7] This would be the factor behind Benjamin Franklin's remark that "like fish, guests begin to smell after three days." Plainly, he felt that his guests were disturbing his arrangements. However, as far as mere face-to-face exposure goes, spending time together leads to liking. Yet, as everyone knows, an increase in liking based on an increase in exposure does not go on indefinitely. For many people there probably comes a critical point at which the exposure is felt as excessive. Much here will depend on both the dynamics of the interactions and the personalities of the individuals involved.

With this we are able to get a picture of how friendship seems to smoothly work its way into a romantic relationship. For romantic partners naturally seek to spend time together. And as they spend time together they will tend to increase their liking for each other. At the same time this mutual liking gives a sense of coming closer to the other person's awareness and therefore of overcoming metaphysical isolation.

Of course, it could be that the romantic partners were already cross-sex friends before their mutual romantic attraction set in. In such a case it might be thought that it was the spending of time together that led to their falling in love. Spending time together can work either to get lovers to be friends or to get friends to be lovers, depending on which they were first. If this is true, then romantic attraction and friendship might not be so very different, for both would be similarly influenced by the liking that results from spending time together. The attempt to overcome metaphysical isolation, it could then be supposed, is the driving force behind both sorts of relationships.

There are, however, several things that make such a view untenable. Not only are there the distinctive features of love mentioned earlier that are lacking in friendship, but spending time together does not seem to increase sexual attraction in the way that it increases liking. That is, sexual attraction is not something that gradually builds up as one spends more and more time with someone. Rather, it is an instantaneous affair that tends to take place in the moment that one first spots the sexually attractive person (though it can take place later when, through liking, one suddenly sees the person in a new way). This is also, as Shakespeare so beautifully shows us, exactly how romantic attraction works. And this should come as no surprise, for as I have tried to argue, sexual attraction lies at the heart of romantic attraction. This, then, strongly suggests that it is not metaphysical isolation (that is, the basis for friendship) that lies behind the pull of romantic attraction. Rather, since it is gender isolation that leads to sexual attraction, and since sexual attraction is the basis of romantic attraction, it seems then that the sense of gender isolation is the ultimate pull of romantic attraction.

But if spending time together does not lead cross-sex friends to fall in love, what then does? The answer to this question should not be too difficult to uncover, for it is the same answer to the question of what leads cross-sex friends to be together in the first place. This answer is sexual attraction. But, someone could ask, if it is sexual attraction that leads cross-sex friends to fall in love, and if sexual attraction happens instantaneously, why is it that cross-sex friends who do fall in love do not always do so instantaneously? Why is it that cross-sex friends are often friends for extended periods (all the while being sexually attracted to each other) before suddenly falling in love?

To understand this, one must start by noting that although love is something that tends to happens swiftly, people can still often decide when to let it happen swiftly. This was my point made earlier about the distinction between romantic attraction and love, and the point of the example of someone who is romantically attracted to another but waiting for a response before letting himself fall fully in love. Although such a view of love may go against popular conceptions—conceptions that see love as something that works beyond our control—simple observation of romantic relationships suggests that people often do choose when to let themselves fall in love. Perhaps we could say that people often climb up in order to wait for the appropriate time to let themselves fall. This is not to say that romantic attraction is fully under our control but only that it is not fully beyond our control.

Consider the real-life example of Sophie, 40 years old, and Simon, 44 years old, work colleagues who had been cross-sex friends for three years before becoming lovers and getting married.[8] For Sophie, Simon had been one of her closest friends, being emotionally supportive while she went through a string of "thrilling but chaotic" relationships. He would even have a drink with her at a bar while she was waiting for one of her new boyfriends to show up and was there as a shoulder to cry on when the affair went awry. Although she described him to her friends as "not very exciting," she explained nevertheless, "I'd go on dates with other men and find myself thinking about him, and once I joked that we should get together. I suppose I was testing the water to judge his reaction. Deep down I knew he already liked me when I made my move." Simon gives his own account, saying, "After a few months of first meeting her I realized I was attracted to her, and as time went by my feelings grew a lot stronger. I'm not the sort of bloke who takes the lead, so I sat back while she went on various dates with other men."

The change came for Sophie when she and Simon were attending their boss's wedding. As Sophie puts it, a change happened quickly: "On that day of the wedding, when everyone around me was saying how lovely he was, I suddenly thought they were right. It was like an epiphany." They were staying at Simon's parents' house for the wedding. The morning after the wedding, says Sophie, "I woke up and thought, 'I am going to ask him to marry me.'" Then, she says, "We were sitting on the bed in his parents' spare room when he kissed me for the first time. If I'm honest, it felt so familiar, and it wasn't a fire-in-the-stomach thing, but it made me very happy. All day I couldn't stop thinking what an amazing person this quiet man had become."

This development came as a surprise for Simon. "I had no idea that Sophie's feelings for me had changed," he says. "Secretly I hoped there might be a future for us, so when she proposed I couldn't have been happier—or more gobsmacked."

Here we have a case of cross-sex friends who were sexually and, it seems, romantically attracted to each other from the start of their relationship, even though they were not openly in love. The reason their attraction seems romantic rather than purely sexual is that both were clearly aware of the other as a possible romantic partner and not just as a sexual partner. Although Sophie described him to her friends as "not very exciting," she nevertheless continued to think about him as she was with other dating partners. Simon, on the other hand, appeared clearer about his attraction to Sophie, saying that within a few months of meeting her he realized he was attracted to her. It seems significant that he said he "realized" he was attracted to her rather than he "became" attracted to her. For this suggests that the attraction was there before he realized it. That his feeling was romantic attraction is indicated by his saying that he hoped there might be a future for them. Therefore, neither of them seemed to be only considering the possibility of becoming, say, sexual friends.

It is interesting that both of them seemed to wait on the other to see how the other would feel. Sophie joked about her and Simon getting together, "testing the water to judge his reaction," while Simon, not being one to take the lead, waited about while Sophie saw other men. The moment when things changed for Sophie was when she suddenly realized how lovely he was. Simon, on the other hand, does not give a specific point at which he fell in love with Sophie. He only says that after a few months he realized he was attracted to her. He does mention that as time went by, his feelings grew a lot stronger. But it is unclear what this means. Since I have argued that romantic attraction is not something that gradually occurs, it might seem that this is a counter-example to my view. For is he not saying, it could be asked, that his romantic feelings for Sophie gradually grew stronger? I think, however, his remark can be understood in another way. For since Simon appears to have been romantically attracted to Sophie right from the start, it was probably frustrating for him to see Sophie going through her "thrilling but chaotic" relationships while being himself regulated to the unexciting sidelines. He also was a shoulder for her to cry on. Thus, he probably spent time consoling her.

Through all this it seems reasonable to suppose that he might have wished more and more that his love toward her could be requited and that he could be the one in the love relationship with her. He does say that he secretly hoped they might have a future together, which sounds much like unrequited love. This seems an entirely plausible interpretation of his statement about his feelings growing stronger over time and, further, is an interpretation that does not refer to romantic attraction occurring gradually. Because of this, my impression is that Simon's romantic attraction occurred swiftly at the beginning of the friendship. He was, however, plainly waiting to see how Sophie felt about him before he let himself fall fully in love with her.

There still remains the question of why Sophie had her epiphany when she did. And here it seems important to note that she was at a wedding when she had this experience. Further, it was shortly after everyone was telling her how lovely Simon was. Finally, she had just been through a series of unsuccessful relationships and also knew that Simon was fond of her. She probably further knew that he was waiting for her to show interest. In this context it is clear that the wedding represented to Sophie, now in her 40s, something that she deeply wanted but was on the verge of never having. What everyone's comments about Simon woke her up to was that Simon was an obvious way of achieving her goal. Even though he was not very exciting, everyone thought he was lovely, and she had toyed with the idea of getting together with him before. Being at a wedding (and with Simon at that) was probably a crucial factor in her falling in love with Simon. This is suggested by the fact that she decided, not to declare her love to Simon or to say that she wanted to be lovers, but rather to ask him straight off to marry her. Clearly, she was a woman in a hurry.

She does not say if she had been three times a bridesmaid or felt herself to be on a par with leftover Christmas cake, but a single woman in her 40s who wants to get married might well begin to worry, especially if she has been through several unsuccessful relationships. At this point she might feel she cannot spend any more time trying to find the right man and so take someone who is readily available, even if he is not very exciting. This common way of thinking was expressed in a figurine I once saw in a joke shop. It was a skeleton wearing a bridal gown slumped to one side on a park bench and covered in cobwebs. On the ground in front of the bench was inscribed the words "Waiting for Mr. Right."

All of this shows the inherent complexity of the notion of falling in love. For much about Sophie's falling in love with Simon is reminiscent of the pragmatic account of choosing a romantic partner that I referred to earlier. There I mentioned the case of a woman who, suddenly realizing all her friends are married, quickly tries to find someone who will marry her so she will not get left behind. In this sort of case, I said that the woman might even try to convince herself that she is in love with man she finds, even though she is not. Sophie's situation is similar to this in that she is also getting older, being unable to find Mr. Right, and watching weddings go by. Because of this she then quickly turns to Simon, for he is someone who is readily available.

Yet her situation is also quite different. For Simon is not someone whom she vaguely remembers and to whom she has no real attraction. She has thought of him previously in a romantic way (while dating her boyfriends). Also, Simon is one of her closest friends and an emotional support. Simon is also romantically attracted to her. Her romantic attraction to him is not overpowering, and even when they kissed for the first time, it was not "a fire-in-the-stomach thing." But romantic attraction, like sexual attraction, can come in varying degrees. Also, many people do not experience romantic love in an emotional way. There being no fire-in-the-stomach, which sounds like a reference to an emotional state, does not therefore show there is no romantic love.

The question then becomes, when Sophie had her epiphany, did she really fall in love with Simon, or did she merely convince herself that she was in love so that she could quickly get married and not get left behind? This is a difficult question to answer. And it may be that neither of these answers is fully satisfactory by itself. For maybe both options apply to her in varying degrees. Maybe she did fall in love with him, though not with the intensity of her earlier thrilling and chaotic relationships. But, with the years and weddings whistling by, she might have come to the conclusion that it was not that essential to have a fire-in-the-stomach romance. Perhaps, she might have begun to think, what was more important was that she had a stable and lasting romantic love (and a marriage to go with it), even if it was with someone who was not very exciting (all the while being aware that Simon was waiting at the sidelines). At this point she might have simply let herself fall in love with Simon. That she did fall in love with him is suggested by her remark, "All day I couldn't stop thinking what an amazing person this quiet man had become." For of course the quiet man had not changed at all. He was "gobsmacked" to discover Sophie's new feelings, but his romantic attraction to her and his hope for a future with her had always been there. Rather, it was Sophie who had changed, for she had let herself fall in love.

THE ALLURE OF ROMANTIC PARTNERS

The fascinating thing about romantic attraction from the standpoint of allure is that it both contains sexual attraction and yet is something more than sexual attraction. Further, these two sorts of attraction are not distinct, for sexual attraction is an integral part of romantic attraction. In addition, romantic attraction frequently takes place alongside the attraction of friendship. This suggests that not only will the allure of a romantic partner differ from the allure of a purely sexual partner, but further that this allure will be affected by the friendship in which it takes place, much like the allure of both cross-sex friends and sexual friends is affected.

Moreover, romantic attraction can take place with or without the partners' ever having had sex, though typically if a romantic relationship is going to persist, it seems that sexual interaction will quickly have to become part of it. It is true that the promise of sex can work to hold newly formed romantic partners together for a certain amount of time, but not indefinitely. This seems to be something that most people are aware of and shows one of the major differences between the allure of the cross-sex friend and the allure of the romantic partner. For in the case of the cross-sex friend, the goal of the allure—the intimate joining of bodies—presents itself to awareness as something that only might happen. In the case of the romantic partner, it presents itself as something that needs to happen, at least if the romantic relationship is to continue. In other words, although not having sex will tend not to have a negative effect on a cross-sex friendship, not having sex will tend to be destructive of a romantic relationship. And here again it is important to remember that having sex does not just refer to sexual intercourse or even just genital interactions, but to any form of intimate baring and caressing. This is why romantic partners who, because of sexual dysfunction or poor health, cannot engage in genital sex can still have their romantic relationships continue. For they can still bare and caress in other ways.

There are, to be sure, many married couples who have been together for years and who show no interest in any form of baring and caressing with each other. Perhaps they even sleep in separate rooms. This, however, does not present a problem for my view, for such couples, I would argue, are not in love. But why are they staying together, year after year, when they have no love for each other? As we all know, there are numerous other nonromantic reasons why people remain in loveless marriages. Perhaps they feel divorce would be an intolerable stigma, or perhaps they remain together for their children's or parents' sake. Or having succumbed to fears of not being able to find another partner, they might simply be too afraid to consider going it alone. Or then again, maybe it is easier to just put one's head down and carry on. How they deal with their sexual desires is another question. Perhaps they resolutely repress them, satisfy them elsewhere, or resign themselves to a life of fantasy and masturbation.

It is therefore evident that the allure of the romantic partner will be complex and many-sided depending on the sort of romantic relationship one is in. If we look at the case of romantic partners who are neither friends nor yet sexual partners, the allure felt here will not be framed in the context of friendship. Allure being thus framed, as we have seen, is what happens in cross-sex and sexual friendships. In this situation, however, the experience of being helplessly drawn will tend to appear by itself without any form of support from the attraction of friendship. In this way it will be like the allure of a stranger, which also lacks the attraction of friendship. In the case of love at first sight, the allure is even more like the allure of a stranger. For here the goal of allure is also unknown. Therefore, as Romeo gazes at Juliet for the first time, falling in love with her while fantasizing the joining of their bodies—his rude hand becoming blessed in hers—he has neither any idea what an exchange of intimacy and concern with her would feel like, nor just what her skin would feel like. For she is essentially an alluring and unnoticing stranger.

Yet the ultimate goal of the allure of the "beloved at first sight" will differ from that in the allure of a stranger. This is because the allure of the romantic partner will contain as its ultimate goal not only the exchange of baring and caressing (the sexual element) with the beloved but also an exchange of psychological vulnerability and care (the psychological and emotional element). It would be a mistake, however, to think that in romantic allure there are two ultimate goals. For, as I have argued, the distinction between these two aspects of romantic attraction is merely theoretical. In the reality of experience, the nonsexual aspect of romantic attraction never appears without the sexual aspect firmly in its midst. As a result, the ultimate goal of romantic attraction is an intimate exchange of vulnerability and care, in all its dimensions, with the beloved.

But what is it about this element of the allure of a "love at first sight" romantic partner that makes it different from that of the allure of a stranger? One of the difficulties about answering this question is that the distinction between these two experiences can be subtle and difficult to draw. This is, of course, because the romantically alluring person who is seen for the first time is much on a par with an alluring stranger. One knows nothing about either save their physical appearance, and, further, the whole basis of the allure in both cases is that of physical appearance. Moreover, the fantasy of oneself in a state of psychological intimacy and concern with the person seems far less precise than the fantasy of oneself in intimate physical contact with her. Because of all this, people often find it difficult to give a precise account of the two types of allure in a way that makes clear their distinction.

An answer, I think, is suggested by something Romeo says when he first sees Juliet. For upon saying how beautiful she is, he immediately adds that she is "Beauty too rich for use." This is a difficult remark to interpret, for how is it that her beauty is too rich for use? One way of understanding this is to compare his situation—being swept away by the allure of a romantically attractive stranger—with that of the allure of a merely sexually attractive stranger. In the case of the sexually attractive stranger, the goal of allure is a sexual interaction with the stranger. Here one is drawn helplessly to the idea of making sexual "use" of the stranger's beauty. One is drawn to the fantasy of encountering the stranger's body through mutual fondling, kissing, and embracing. All of this can be said to be a way in which the stranger's beauty is put to (sexual) use.

What Romeo is saying, then, is that Juliet's beauty is too rich to be simply used in this way. But this cannot mean that he is not allured to a bodily joining with her. For he immediately fantasizes touching her hand and upon meeting her not only takes her hand but does what he can to get a kiss from her. This is also sexual use. What he means in saying this, then, is that a sexual encounter with her cannot make use of all her beauty. Her beauty is too multifaceted for just sexual use. How else then can he use her beauty? The answer is he can engage her in an exchange of psychological vulnerability and care. This is made plain in their first encounter. For what he does here is to make himself vulnerable to her by suggesting that his hand is unworthy to touch her, possibly profaning the holy shrine that is her. Why does he do this? He is, of course, being flirtatious and ultimately trying to get a kiss. But he is also doing this so that she may respond to his vulnerability with care. And this is exactly what she does. Showing concern and care for the state he has put himself in, she replies, "Good pilgrim, you do wrong your hand too much" (though at another level she is coyly trying to avoid giving a kiss). He then kisses her, saying her lips have purged his sin (taken care of his vulnerability). She replies, "Then have my lips the sin that they have took," suggesting her own vulnerability, which he then offers to care for by taking back the sin with another kiss.

This exchange of psychological vulnerability and care is thus interwoven with hand-holding, attempts to get a kiss, and finally a kiss. In other words, it is done with an exchange of baring and caressing. It is this psychological component, inexorably entangled with the sexual component, that is the ultimate goal of romantic allure. It is what we feel ourselves being helplessly drawn toward when we feel the allure of a romantically attractive person. However, because the romantically attractive person is in this case essentially an alluring stranger, it will be difficult to draw a precise line between the two sorts of allure. This is because the alluring stranger can also present herself to awareness as nearly romantically alluring. Here she can also enter one's awareness as beauty too rich for use. In this case one gazes upon her, nearly overwhelmed by her allure, invaded by the sense that even sexual union with her would not completely fulfill the goal of the allure. In this instance the goal of the allure can hover somewhere between that of an alluring stranger and that of an alluring romantic partner.

This is the experience captured in the declaration "I think I'm in love!" which is sometimes uttered upon seeing an alluring stranger. The reason the declaration is "I think I'm in love!" rather than simply "I'm in love!" is precisely that the goal of the allure hovers between the intimate joining of bodies and the intimate joining of bodies blended with an intimate exchange of psychological vulnerability and care. Consequently, the one making the declaration cannot say for certain he is in love.

One man in his 40s with whom I discussed this went even further. When I asked him to describe his experience of falling in love, he laughed and replied, "I fall in love 20 times a day." The women he fell in love with each day were the sexually or rather romantically attractive strangers he passed in the street. This was, he assured me, romantic attraction, as he would have loved to have had each one of them as a romantic partner. What stopped him from attempting to pursue these attractive strangers was simply the impracticability of acting on every such attraction.

In the case of romantic partners who have had romantic interactions, both physical and psychological, this goal of allure remains the same, with the exception that it transforms into something more concrete. This is because, in this case, the goal of allure has already been achieved. It is this feature of already having achieved the goal, it will be recalled, that distinguishes the allure of sexual friends from the allure of cross-sex friends. In this case, the goal is simply having sex. The fact that sexual friends have already had sex while cross-sex friends have not means that the goal of allure for sexual friends presents itself in a more concrete form than it does for cross-sex friends. This is because the sexual friend's sexual interactions remain in her awareness to be taken up in subsequent experiences of allure. Because of this, the sexual friend knows full well what she is being allured toward in a way that the cross-sex friend does not. In this way, too, the allure of a person with whom one has romantically interacted is different from the allure of a romantically attractive person with whom one has not thus interacted. For here, too, the previous interactions remain in one's awareness as ready material for the subsequent fantasies of allure. This means that the lover who has shared intimacies and care with her partner, has kissed, held, and had sex with her partner, will have more definite material from which the ultimate goal of the allure can be constructed. Since this material also comes from previous experience with the romantic partner, it gives the goal of allure a sense of being actually attainable. This is in contrast to the romantic allure, whose goal is not constructed of previous romantic experience with the beloved. For in this case there is a sense of the romantic interaction being only potentially attainable.

Nevertheless, in both cases the prominent feature of the fantasy of allure will here be an intimate joining of bodies. For this is what people typically refer to in describing their experience of romantic attraction to their partner. Where the exchange of psychological vulnerability and care come into the allure is through the meanings that the images of these bodily joinings can take. Therefore, the fantasized image will not simply be a naked embrace, or the kissing of a vulva, but rather "embracing me in a way that shows he deeply cares" or "kissing my vulva in a caring and loving way."

Naturally, in the case of someone who has already had romantic interactions with the beloved, such fantasies will present themselves as something actually attainable. This is in contrast to the fantasies in the allure of the "beloved at first sight." In this case, the lover has no direct experience upon which to base his or her fantasized images of sexual interaction with the beloved. These must be simply guessed at or imported and adapted from elsewhere. Because the lover who has already romantically interacted with the beloved will not be at a deficit in this way, his or her sense of being drawn will contain a directional sharpness. That is, the feeling of being drawn toward a romantic interaction with his or her romantic partner will here be bathed in a sharp and lucid sense of being swept toward the goal of the allure. This, again, is supported by what we know about the nature of sexual fantasies and how they tend to be firmly tied to real events.

A distinction between these two instances of romantic allure can also be observed in their elements of helplessness. This mirrors a similar distinction I referred to earlier, namely the distinction between helplessness as it appears in the allure of the cross-sex friend and as it appears in the allure of the sexual friend. There I pointed out that just as there is an element of helplessness in allure, so is there an element of helplessness in having sex. In allure the helplessness attends the sense of being drawn toward the sexually attractive person, while in many forms of sexual interaction the helplessness appears in such places as nearly automated actions, the compelling feature of fore-pleasure, the sense of the inevitability of orgasm and, with the male, of ejaculation, the autonomous character of peak pleasure, and the waves of pulsation following orgasm. These experiences, all of which can take place in having sex, seem to appear beyond our control and so create a sense of being helpless before them.

Most if not all of these instances of helplessness will thus have occurred in relationships that involve a sexual relationship. This includes the romantic relationship in which the partners have had sex. Now, since allure exists within a romantic relationship independently of the partners' having had sex, the sense of helplessness is already there before sex takes place. However, once sexual interaction is added to the relationship, new experiences of helplessness (those experienced within sexual encounters) are also added. Here, then, we have a situation similar to that of the experience of helplessness in sexual friendships. For sexual friends also experience helplessness in both their allure to one another and their sexual interactions.

In discussing this doubling of helplessness in the experience of sexual friends, I noted that since the sexual experiences of helplessness share much in common with the helplessness component of allure, the sense of helplessness that occurs in sex can easily merge with the helplessness of allure, thus intensifying it. This is precisely what happens in the case of the romantic allure one has to a sexual partner. For here there is also both sexual attraction and sexual interaction. However, the situation here differs in an important way. This is because the sexual attraction that takes place is part of romantic attraction, which is not the case in sexual attraction to a sexual friend. The ultimate goal of allure in the allure of a sexual friend is the fantasy of the intimate union of two bodies. This goal is also there in romantic attraction. But as I tried to show, it is inexorably entangled with the component of psychological intimacy and care.

Thus, what I am allured to by my romantic partner is presented in a fantasy of sexual union that carries with it meanings of psychological union through an intimate exchange of vulnerability and care. Because these meanings center around psychological vulnerability and care, and because vulnerability is connected to the idea of helplessness, we can see then that a third layer of helplessness works its way into the allure of the romantic partner. First, there is the helplessness of being drawn. Second, there is the helplessness that appears in the memories of the sexual encounters. Third, there is the helplessness that appears in the memories of being psychologically and emotionally vulnerable during earlier romantic interactions. And again, just as the first two instances of helplessness will tend to merge into an intensified sense of helplessness, so will the third instance easily join in. I am not saying that these different appearances of helplessness will be lucidly discernible for anyone in the throes of allure, but only that there will tend to be a sense of the multiple origins of the intensified feeling of being helplessly drawn to the beloved. This account helps to explain the fact that once one has tasted the beloved, so to speak, as a romantic partner, one is even more powerfully, and thus more helplessly, drawn toward him or her.

This is nicely portrayed in Romeo's second encounter with Juliet, when he sees her at her window in the night. For at this point, having already held her hand and kissed her, he has had a taste of her delights. In his first viewing of her, he is clearly enthralled with her. But in the second encounter, he cannot contain himself. The first time he sees her, she teaches the torches to burn bright and he fantasizes touching her hand. But at the second sighting, she is the sun itself. Seeing her lean her cheek upon her hand, he fantasizes being a glove on her hand in order that he could touch her cheek. His helplessness in being drawn to her is revealed in his compulsion to speak to her from his hiding spot, despite being in a dangerous situation: "I will answer" and "Shall I hear more, or shall I speak at this?" he says to himself before at last impulsively calling out to her.

This already complex picture of the allure of the romantic partner becomes even more complex when the romantic partner is also a friend. For here, in addition to the allure that works on the lover, there is the attraction of friendship. These, of course, are separate experiences. Nonetheless, they will have a tendency to blend together as they interact in drawing the romantic partners together. In this case, the friendship will affect the allure much as it did in the case of sexual friendship. It, too, will tend to create a sharp and lucid feeling of being drawn unmistakably toward to the other person. Here the friendship will also create a warm and supportive atmosphere in which the allure does its work. Further, I also suggested that friendship itself can contain the notion of helplessness. Though not continually present as an aspect of friendship, it nevertheless appears as being related to the idea of well-wishing and well-doing. For these are both forms of care, and care is especially appropriate for someone who is in need of care, or, in other words, helpless.

Because, however, the friendship happens together with a romantic allure rather than just a sexual allure, the friendship will tend to exert an effect on the allure. The reason for this is that romantic allure has more in common with friendship than does purely sexual allure. This is because while the goal of sexual allure is simply the joining of one's body with that of the other person, the goal of romantic allure is not only bodily joining, but also the exchange of psychological vulnerability and care. This means that it has something in common with friendship. For the attraction of friendship also involves an exchange of psychological elements, namely, the psychological elements that comprise the liking of friendship. As I pointed out earlier in this chapter, romantic attraction is not simply a more intense version of the liking of friendship, for the two forms of attraction differ in basic ways. This, however, does not mean they share nothing in common. For regardless of their differences, they are both still forms of interpersonal attraction that necessarily are concerned with psychological elements. It is even probably because of this commonality that many people fail to distinguish clearly between them, seeing romantic love as merely a more intense form of friendship.

Because, then, romantic attraction and friendship share this feature, friendship is able to give further impetus to the allure of the romantic partner. Thus, as I watch my romantic partner I feel myself allured by her to an intimate exchange of vulnerability and care, in all its dimensions. This intimate exchange appears in my fantasy of a sexual interaction with her where the sexual activities carry meanings that point to psychological dimensions of vulnerability and care. Since, however, she is also my friend, I am at the same time in a relationship of mutual liking with her. This mutual liking involves companionship or the enjoyment of her company simply for the sake of being with her.

This enjoyment of her company for its own sake is naturally different from the enjoyment of her company for the sake of an exchange of psychological vulnerability and care. But they are nevertheless similar so far as both are concerned with psychological aspects. Because of this, my friendship with her acts as a support for the romantic allure she sends out to me. For both are instances of moving toward her. Just as her romantic allure magnetically pulls me to her, so does my liking for her as a friend make me seek out her company.

These attractions are to different things and thus do not attract me to her in the same way at the same time. But there is no need for them to do so. In one moment I am allured to her romantically: the femaleness of her skin and the slender curve of her neck, along with the meanings of mutual vulnerability and care that my caressing her would involve, all press themselves forward in my awareness, alluring me toward her as my romantic partner. But then, in the next moment I see her eyes sparkle with the liking of friendship. In that instance I suddenly am filled with my liking for her as my friend: wishing her well and wanting to help her, being aware of her similar wishes toward me, and enjoying her company for just its own sake. In this instance, her romantic attractiveness has not disappeared. It is still there, but it slips into the background as her appearance as a friend pushes forward to take the central place in my awareness. This oscillation between the two forms of awareness can sometimes be observed in romantic partners when, in the midst of a conversation or some shared activity of friendship, one of the them suddenly focuses on the other in a different way, taking his hand, kissing him, or otherwise displaying affection. What often happens in this situation is that the romantic attraction has suddenly pressed itself to the fore, and the person experiencing the attraction responds to this by bringing her body together with his; that is, brings about the goal of the allure he or she feels toward his or her partner.

In this sense, having a romantic partner who is also a friend is much like having a cross-sex friend. For in the case of the cross-sex friend, there is also both allure and friendship. In fact, the heterosexual romantic partner who is also a friend *is* a cross-sex friend. Consequently, the experiential mechanisms in cross-sex friendships that I discussed in Chapter Three—the manner in which friendship provides a context for the allure to take place—will also be at work in romantic friendships. There is, however, a basic difference at this point between the cross-sex friend and the romantic partner. This is because in the allure of the cross-sex friend, there is no reference to psychological elements. There is, of course, reference to psychological elements in the friendship component of cross-sex friendships, but not in the allure component, which only concerns the joining of bodies.

But in the allure of the romantic partner, there is more than just a joining of bodies, there is also a reference to a psychological element, namely, to the exchange of psychological vulnerability and care. This means that within the romantic relationship to someone who is also a friend, there appear two references to psychological elements: one in the exchange of psychological vulnerability and care, and one in the mutual liking of friendship. These are different types of psychological elements, for friendship and romantic attraction are quite distinct. Nonetheless, they still both refer to concerns with psychological dimensions and so at least share that in common. When both romantic attraction and friendship occur toward the same person, this similarity between the two types of attraction works to build a bridge between them, creating an overall sense of attraction to the other person.

Although this might sound as though it would increase the allure of the romantic partner by increasing the sense of being drawn, this is not what seems to happen. That is, it does not appear that romantic partners who are friends are more powerfully allured to each other than are, say, lovers at first sight. My impression is that what happens instead is that the allure acquires a sense of familiarity. This is because the goal of romantic allure is the exchange of vulnerability and care in all of its dimensions, one of which is the dimension of psychological vulnerability and care. This psychological dimension, of which the lover is aware, associates easily with the liking of friendship. Since one has a sense of familiarity with one's friends, this sense of familiarity is then effortlessly imparted to the romantic allure, providing it with a context of familiarity in which the allure can take place.

This is how Sophie, who is both friend and lover with Simon, describes her first kiss with Simon: "If I'm honest, it felt so familiar." But where did this sense of familiarity come from? It could not have come from an earlier kiss, for this was their first. The answer, it seems, is that it came from the romantic allure that brought her to kiss him. For in that allure there would be the fantasy of a kiss surrounded by the psychological exchange of vulnerability and care. This would have a natural connection to her feelings of friendship for Simon, for being his friend, she would have a sense of familiarity toward him. Because of this natural connection, her feelings of familiarity toward him would transfer seamlessly to the romantic allure she feels for him. Interestingly, she also says, "and it wasn't a fire-in-the-stomach thing." But I do not think this has much to do with the sense of familiarity. That it does not is also suggested by her use of "and" to join this clause to the one about familiarity. For in connecting the two ideas in this way, it as if they are not necessarily connected. I rather think that the lack of "fire-in-the-stomach" comes from the fact that she herself finds him not very exciting.

Yet there is no reason why romantic partners who are also friends cannot have "fire-in-the-stomach" when engaged in their mutual caresses. In other words, being friends and lovers is quite compatible with feeling passionate excitement toward each other, though much will depend naturally on the strength of the romantic attraction. One thing that can be said is that, as mentioned earlier, without such a friendship it is unlikely that the romantic relationship will be a happy one. Thus, for a romantic relationship to turn out so right, even being in love forever will not really help unless they are also friends forever.

SIX

With the Help of Helplessness

At the beginning of this book I pointed out that sexual attraction plays a major role in most people's lives. There I showed how people around us are continually presented to our awareness in terms of their sexual attractiveness. Having now reached the end of this inquiry, the implications of this widespread sexual attraction become apparent. For it has now been shown that at the heart of sexual attraction lies the experience of allure, an experience that consists of the sense of being helplessly drawn to an intimate physical joining with another person. Moreover, allure is at work in a diverse range of relationships. This means that throughout our daily encounters with other people—those we pass in the street, work colleagues, classmates, friends, romantic partners, and others—we are continuously confronted with a sense of helplessness. This is the helplessness that arises immediately upon noticing any sexual attractiveness the person presents to us. This can be experienced as irresistible, barely noticeable, or anywhere in between. In all cases, some degree of a sense of helplessness mingles in our awareness as we undergo the presence of the sexually attractive person. Of course, there are also the other features of allure, namely, the sense of being drawn and the sexual fantasy of what one is being drawn toward. But these are also both deeply tied to the sense of helplessness, for in being drawn we are helplessly drawn and in having fantasies appear to us, we are helpless before them: they appear of their own accord. This is their spontaneous and autochthonic quality.

What makes helplessness stand out is that it challenges our sense of free will. Free will refers to the idea that human beings are not mechanically determined in their behavior, thoughts, and preferences, but instead can act, think, and decide according to their own choices. Most people accept that our choices guide our actions, but the determinist view is that even if our choices guide our actions, the choices themselves are not really free because they themselves are ultimately caused by events beyond our control. Proponents of free will, however, argue that even though other events clearly influence our choices, in the end nothing forces us to make one choice rather than another. Each choice is freely chosen and we could have always done otherwise. To be sure, we are limited by our physical constitution and by our environment, but within those limitations, according to the idea of free will, it is our decisions alone that guide our actions and thoughts. The question of whether we have free will is one that has been much discussed by philosophers and there is little agreement about its answer. But whether or not we have free will, the fact remains that we do have a sense of free will whenever we make a choice. For in choosing one alternative over another, people typically sense that they had a genuine choice and that they could have chosen the alternative if they had so wanted.

It is just this sense of free will that becomes challenged when the experience of helplessness appears. For in being helpless before the sexually attractive person, we feel our sense of autonomy begin to slip away. It is almost as if the sexually attractive person sets off something within us that disables our ability to look the other way, to continue our chain of thought, or to proceed in the direction we were going. Of course, each person will experience this disablement in his or her own way. Also, the degree to which one responds in this way will depend on how sexually attractive one finds the other person. In all cases, however, if we are under the sway of the other person's allure, then our own helplessness before him or her will make itself heard. It is important to see, however, that nothing in this sense of helplessness makes us act in ways beyond our sense of free choice, for the helplessness we experience in allure never makes us do anything. What happens in allure is simply that we experience a sense of helplessness.

Of course, allure is not the only place where we can have this experience. The sense of helplessness can occur in numerous situations throughout our lives. However, there are few everyday human relationships where the sense of helplessness is an essential feature of the relationship. It is noteworthy that one other common relationship where the experience of helplessness comes to the fore is the parent–infant relationship. For here the infant is quite aware of its own helplessness before the parent. This is significant, because as I have tried to show, allure has its origins in the infant's relation to the opposite-sex parent. It is altogether likely, then, that this early experience of helplessness is the template for the later experience that manifests itself in the structure of allure. The helplessness of this early stage is disguised and reborn in the older person as the helplessness of sexual attraction.

Now, because this experience of helplessness calls our sense of free will into question, various meanings will tend to surround the idea of free choice. One is the idea that sexual attraction is not something that is up for us to decide. Rather, through allure it snatches hold of us and forces us to notice the sexually attractive person, orientating ourselves toward him or her while fantasies of intimacy with the person seep into our awareness. Of course, one can say to oneself, "I'm not going to let this person's sexual attractiveness affect me!" and then do what one can to send one's thoughts off in another direction. But by then, it is already too late. That is, the allure has already done its work, which is precisely why one must make an effort to send one's thoughts off in another direction. If the allure had not grabbed hold of and infiltrated one with a sense of helplessness, then there would be no need to fight against it. Further, in thus fighting against the allure, one has already taken notice of and orientated oneself toward the sexually attractive person. It is just this notice of and orientation toward the person that, in such a case, makes someone then attempt to "not let the person's sexual attractiveness affect me."

With this discovery we have come upon a peculiar feature of sexual attraction. This is the fact that sexual attraction, through allure's element of helplessness, sets us on a course to other people whether we like it or not. In other words, it is a way of drawing us toward others beyond the sense of having freely chosen to do so. Other forms of interpersonal relations also bring us together with other people. Liking, friendship, affiliation, and so forth are all instances of where we seek out other people. But such relationships are not typically instances in which we feel ourselves helplessly drawn. It is true that these sorts of ties to other people are referred to as forms of interpersonal attraction. Consequently, this may create the impression that they are also, like sexual attraction, forms of attraction and, as a result, will contain a similar experience of helplessness. But as I mentioned in the first chapter, the term "interpersonal attraction" is normally used to refer to any form of positive attitude toward other people, and the idea of a positive attitude does not carry with it the idea of helplessness. Sexual attraction is usually also a type of positive attitude toward other people, but it does contain the idea of helplessness. This is one of the major distinctions between it and other forms of interpersonal attraction (other than romantic attraction, which is based on sexual attraction).

Someone could, however, question the idea of whether sexual attraction is inherently a positive attitude toward other people. For although sexual attraction is often a positive experience, there are times when someone might find sexual attraction to be unwanted or a burden. In Chapter Three, for example, I referred to the fact that some people feel the sexual attraction they have to their cross-sex friend to be a burden or worrisome. Because of such experiences it might be felt that there is nothing essentially positive about the attitude of sexual attraction, for here seems to be a case where sexual attraction is felt as unpleasant.

A little reflection, however, should show that it is not the sexual attraction itself that is felt to be unpleasant, but rather the dissonance created by conflicts the person has concerning the sexual attraction. Thus, as I said in Chapter Three, the person who finds his sexual attraction toward his cross-sex friend to be worrying finds it that way because he has other concerns that conflict with the sexual attraction. He might, for example, feel guilty or embarrassed about the attraction because he believes it is inappropriate to have such feelings, or he might be concerned that it could lead to an unwanted sexual relationship. But this is nothing inherently unpleasant about the sexual attraction he feels. Rather, the unpleasantness appears only because his attraction clashes with his other goals.

Returning now to the idea of helplessness, it should be noted that there will probably be unusual cases of other forms of interpersonal attraction where something like helplessness seems to take place. In such cases, however, it is not the essence of these relationships that one feels helplessly drawn within them. It is not, for example, an essential part of friendship that friends feel helplessly drawn to one another. Friendships are rather interpersonal relationships where each friend, with a full sense of free choice, actively seeks out the other.

This is not to deny that someone might, because of a pressing psychological state or because of unusual circumstances, feel helplessly drawn to his or her friend. But were this to be a consistent and core feature of his or her relation to the other person, then the question would immediately arise as to whether the relationship was merely a friendship because there is nothing in the reported features of friendship that suggests a sense of helplessness before the friend. Were a person consistently to feel helplessly drawn toward his or her friend, this would be a hint that a sexual element was somehow at play, which is altogether possible. But this would not show that helplessness was an essential or even typical element of friendship, but only that one can have both friendship and sexual attraction toward the same person. This is what was shown in the chapters on cross-sex and sexual friendships. And the same would hold for other interpersonal relations.

Further, not only does sexual attraction set us on a course to others in a state of helplessness, but it also sends us on this course toward those of a specific gender—in heterosexual attraction it is the opposite gender, in homosexual attraction it is the same gender. Moreover, the gender of those it pulls us helplessly toward is not incidental. Rather, it lies at the very nucleus of the helplessness we feel. Thus, in an instance of the helplessness of allure, we do not simply feel helplessness before another person, but helplessness before a male or female person. The maleness or femaleness is crucial here, because it is this that generates the helplessness by being the foundation of that which allures us.

In this way, sexual attraction does not wait upon our pleasure, but as soon as the sexually attractive person of the right gender appears, it does what it can to set us in motion toward that person. I argued at the outset of this study that sexual attraction shows its decisive role in our lives by typically leading us to those who become our sexual, romantic, or lifelong partners. Since it is in these relationships that most people's well-being lies, then, in a way, sexual attraction does not wait upon our own efforts to find our own well-being but, with the help of helplessness, sends us there by itself.

Notes

ONE: INTERPERSONAL ATTRACTION AND SEXUAL ATTRACTION

1. Vigil, 2007.
2. Cialdini, 1984.
3. Montoya and Horton, 2013.
4. Cook and McHenry, 1978.
5. Nikolajeva, 2014, p. 2. (Quotation in the text is my translation.)
6. Collins, 2000; Feinberg et al., 2005.
7. Collins and Missing, 2003.
8. Feinberg et al., 2005.
9. Borkowska and Pawlowski, 2011.
10. Pollick et al., 2005.
11. Morris et al., 2013.
12. Flora, 2010.
13. Advertisement, 2011.
14. Nisbett and Wilson, 1977.
15. Feingold, 1991.
16. Montoya et al., 2008; Morry, 2005, 2007.
17. Walster, et al., 1966.
18. Muirstein, 1972; White, 1980.
19. Berscheid et al., 1971.
20. Vātsyāyana, 1994, p. 103.
21. Burley, 1983.
22. Kenrick et al., 1993; Poulsen et al., 2012.

23. Marrow, 1997, p. 143.
24. Poulsen et al., 2012.
25. Poulsen et al., 2012.
26. Hatfield and Berscheid, 1974.
27. Hensley, 1994.
28. Hensley 1994; Nettle, 2002.
29. Darwin, 1871; Madrigal and Kelly, 2007.
30. Feinman and Gill, 1978.
31. Aristotle, 1941a, p. 1083.
32. Astra and Singg, 2000.
33. Crouse and Mehrabian, 1977.
34. Glassenberg et al., 2010.
35. Dixon, 1983; Krafft-Ebing, 1997.
36. Cialdini, 1984; Langlois et al., 2000.
37. Hatfield and Sprecher, 1986.
38. Kinsey et al., 1948, 1953.
39. Singh, 2006.
40. Giles, 2004.
41. Maner et al., 2003.
42. New York Times Magazine, 2000.
43. Hicks and Leitenberg, 2001.
44. Maltz and Boss, 1997.
45. Doskoch, 1995.
46. Hicks and Leitenberg, 2001.
47. Penton-Voak and Perrett, 2000.
48. Freud, 1900, 1905a.
49. Freud, 1905b; Keiser, 1953.
50. Miller, 1969.
51. Wiszewska et al., 2007.
52. Bereczkei et al., 2004.
53. Bereczkei et al., 2002.
54. Freese and Meland, 2000.
55. Wiggins et al., 1968.
56. Little et al., 2003.
57. Geher, 2012.
58. Hinz, 1989; Little et al., 2003.
59. Little et al., 2011.
60. Pelham et al., 2005.
61. Glassenberg et al., 2010.
62. Slater et al., 1998; Langlois et al., 1987.
63. Symons, 1979.

64. Bomba and Siqueland, 1983; Kuhl, 1991.
65. Rubenstein et al., 1999.

TWO: EXCHANGING GLANCES

1. Argyle, 1988; Knapp et al., 2013.
2. Goffman, 1959.
3. Williams, 1944.
4. Maltz and Boss, 1997, p. 48.
5. Argyle and Cook, 1976.
6. Hess, 1965.
7. Bull and Shead, 1979; Stass and Willis, 1967; Tomlinson et al., 1978.
8. Bull and Shead, 1979, Stass and Willis, 1967; Tomlinson et al., 1978.
9. Glassenberg et al., 2010.
10. Perrett et al., 1998.
11. Dixson et al., 2007, 2010.
12. Sartre, 1956.
13. Wilson et al., 1963.
14. Tlachi-Lópeza et al., 2012.
15. Lisk and Baron, 1982.
16. Little et al., 2014.
17. Hall and Van de Castle, 1966.
18. Schredl et al., 2009.
19. Domhoff, 2003; Hall 1951; Lortie-Lussier et al., 2000.
20. Schredl, 2012.
21. Freud, 1900.
22. Hall, 1963.
23. Schneider and Domhoff, 2014.
24. Schneider and Domhoff, 2014.
25. Schneider and Domhoff, 2014.
26. Schneider and Domhoff, 2014.
27. Spock, 1967.
28. Reddy, 2010.
29. Chivers et al., 2004.
30. Keller, 2007.

THREE: JUST FRIENDS

1. Paine, 1969.
2. Seiden and Bart, 1975.
3. Lazarsfeld and Merton, 1954.

4. Rubin, 1985.
5. Aristotle, 1941b, p. 1386.
6. Honneth, 2013.
7. Beer, 2001.
8. Confucius, 2001, p. 30.
9. Lu, 2010.
10. Demir and Doğan, 2013.
11. Rubin, 1985, pp. 56–57.
12. Parten, 1932; Rubin et al, 2006.
13. Jacklin and Maccoby, 1978.
14. Fouts et al., 2013; Munroe and Romney, 2006; Whiting and Edwards, 1988.
15. Maccoby, 1990.
16. Maccoby, 1990; Rubin et al., 2006; Rose and Rudolph, 2006.
17. Rubin, 1980.
18. Underwood, 2003.
19. Rose and Rudolph, 2006.
20. Benenson and Christakos, 2003.
21. Bell, 1981, p. 50.
22. Hazan and Diamond, 2000.
23. Rubin, 1985.
24. Giles, 2010.
25. Cicero, 1887, p. 57.
26. Myers et al., 2005.
27. Xiaohe and Whyte, 1990.
28. Bell, 1981, p. 127.
29. Bell, 1981, p. 127.
30. Afifi and Faulkner, 2000.
31. Willis, 2014.
32. Gilligan, 1982.
33. Afifi and Faulkner, 2000; Bleske-Rechek et al., 2012; Reeder, 2000.
34. O'Meara, 1989.
35. Werking, 1997.
36. Rose, 1985.
37. Harvey, 2004, p. 164.
38. Monsour, 2002.
39. Halatsis and Christakis, 2009.
40. Halatsis and Christakis, 2009.
41. Rubin, 1985, p. 162.
42. Kaggwa, 2013.

43. Rubin, 1985; Monsour, 2002.
44. Afifi and Faulkner, 2000.
45. Bell, 1981.
46. Monsour, 1992.
47. Bisson and Levine, 2009.
48. Miller et al., 2014.
49. Bleske-Rechek et al., 2012.
50. Bleske-Rechek et al., 2012.
51. Bell, 1981; Halatsis and Christakis, 2009.
52. Bratman, 1987.
53. Halatsis and Christakis, 2009; Rawlins, 1982; Werking, 1997.
54. Halatsis and Christakis, 2009, p. 920.
55. Halatsis and Christakis, 2009, p. 920.

FOUR: MORE THAN JUST FRIENDS

1. Bradac, 1983.
2. Rawlins, 1982.
3. O'Meara, 1989, p. 530.
4. Conley et al., 2012.
5. Levine and Mongeau, 2010.
6. Weaver et al., 2011.
7. Erlandsson et al., 2012.
8. McGee, 2011.
9. Stephens, 2010, p. 84.
10. Paul et al., 2000.
11. VanderDrift et al., 2010.
12. Mongeau et al., 2013.
13. Mongeau et al., 2013, p. 39.
14. Giles, 2004.
15. Rubin, 1985, pp. 151–152.
16. Werking, 1997, p. 30.
17. Paul et al., 2000.
18. Hansen et al., 2014.
19. Hupka, 1981.
20. Afifi and Faulkner, 2000.
21. Levine and Mongeau, 2010.
22. Owen et al., 2013.
23. Anonymous, 2011.
24. Bisson and Levine, 2009.

25. Erlandsson et al., 2012.
26. Owen et al., 2013.
27. Millet, 2003, pp. 177–178.
28. Cleary, 1999.
29. Barker, 2007, p. 23.
30. Weinberg et al., 1995, p. 7.
31. Freud, 1905a, p. 208.
32. Vātsyāyana, 1994, p. 166.
33. Zilbergeld, 1999.
34. Zilbergeld, 1999, p. 203.

FIVE: IT TURNED OUT SO RIGHT

1. Giles, 2004; Hatfield and Berscheid, 1974.
2. Shakespeare, 2003.
3. Nietzsche, 2007. (Quotation in the text is my translation.)
4. Hatfield and Walster 1981, p. 9.
5. Conlon, 1995, pp. 297–298.
6. Festinger et al., 1950.
7. Ebbeson et al., 1976.
8. Tucker, 2008.

References

Advertisement (2011, June 7). *Banyule & Nillumbik Weekly: Your Community Voice*, 17.

Afifi, W. A., and Faulkner, S. L. (2000). On being "just friends": The frequency and impact of sexual activity in cross-sex friendships. *Journal of Social and Personal Relationships, 17S*, 205–222.

Anonymous. (2011). FWB. Reader comment on A. Ben-Zeév (2011). In the name of love: Friends with benefits. *Psychology Today*. Retrieved October 13, 2014, from http://www.psychologytoday.com/blog/in-the-name-love/201109/friends-benefits/comments

Argyle, M. (1988). *Bodily communication* (2nd ed.). New York: Routledge.

Argyle, M., and Cook, M. (1976). *Gaze and mutual gaze.* Cambridge: Cambridge University Press.

Aristotle. (1941a). *Nichomachean ethics* (W. D. Ross, Trans.). In R. Mckeon (Ed.), *The basic works of Aristotle* (pp. 935–1226). New York: Random House.

Aristotle. (1941b). Rhetorica (W. R. Roberts, Trans.). In R. McKeon, (Ed.), *The basic writings of Aristotle* (pp. 1325–1451). New York: Random House.

Astra, R. L., and Singg, S. (2000). The role of self-esteem in affiliation. *Journal of Psychology: Interdisciplinary and Applied, 34*, 15–22.

Barker, M. (2007). *Review of the nature of sexual desire* by James Giles. *Culture, Health and Sexuality, 9*, 211–213.

Beer, B. (2001). Anthropology of friendship. In N. J. Smelser and P. B. Baltes (Eds.), *International encyclopedia of the social and behavioral sciences* (pp. 5805–5808). Kidlington, UK: Elsevier.

Bell, R. (1981). *Worlds of friendship*. Beverly Hills: Sage.

Benenson, J. F., and Christakos, A. (2003). The greater fragility of females' versus males' closest same-sex friendships. *Child Development, 74*, 1123–1129.

Bereczkei, T., Gyuris, P., and Weisfeld, G. E. (2004). Sexual imprinting in human mate choice. *Proceedings of the Royal Society London, B, 271*, 1129–1134.

Bereczkei, T., Gyuris, P., Koves, P., and Bernath, L. (2002). Homogamy, similarity, and genetic imprinting: Parental influence on mate choice preferences. *Personality and Individual Differences, 33*, 677–690.

Berscheid, E., Dion, K., Walster, E., and Walster, G. W. (1971). Physical attractiveness and dating choice: A test of the matching hypothesis. *Journal of Experimental Psychology, 7*, 173–189.

Bisson, M. A., and Levine, T. R. (2009). Negotiating a friends with benefits relationship. *Archives of Sexual Behavior, 38*, 66–73.

Bleske-Rechek, A., Somers, E., Micke, C., Erickson, L., Matteson, L., et al. (2012). Benefit or burden? Attraction in cross-sex friendship. *Journal of Social and Personal Relationships, 29*, 569–596.

Bomba, P. C., and Siqueland, E. R. (1983). The nature and structure of infant form categories. *Journal of Experimental Child Psychology, 35*, 294–328.

Borkowska, B., and Pawlowski, B. (2011). Female voice frequency in the context of dominance and attractiveness perception. *Animal Behaviour, 82*, 55–59.

Bradac, J. J. (1983). The language of lovers, flovers, and friends: Communicating in social and personal relationships. *Journal of Language and Social Psychology, 2*, 141–162.

Bratman, M. (1987). *Intention, plans, and practical reason.* Cambridge, MA: Harvard University Press.

Bull, R., and Shead, G. (1979). Pupil dilation, sex of stimulus, and age and sex of observer. *Perceptual and Motor Skills, 49*, 27–30.

Burley, N. (1983). The meaning of assortative mating. *Ethology and Sociobiology, 4*, 191–203.

Chivers, M. L., Rieger, G., Latty, E., and Bailey, M. J. (2004). A sex difference in the specificity of sexual arousal. *Psychological Science, 15*, 736–744.

Cialdini, R. B. (1984). *Influence.* New York: William Morrow.

Cicero, M. T. (1887). De amicitia (on friendship). In A. P. Peabody (Ed. and Trans.) *Ethical writings of Cicero: De officiis; de senectute; de amicitia, and Scipio's dream* (pp. 1–71). Boston: Little, Brown, and Company.

Cleary, T. (Trans.). (1999). *Sex, health, and long life: Manuals of Taoist practice*. Boston: Shambala.

Collins, S. A. (2000). Male voices and women's choices. *Animal Behaviour, 60,* 773–780.

Collins S. A., and Missing, C. (2003). Vocal and visual attractiveness are related in women. *Animal Behaviour, 65,* 997–1004.

Confucius. (2001). *The analects* (A. Waley, Trans.). New York: Everyman's Library.

Conley, T. D., Ziegler, A., Moors, A. C., Matsick, J. L., and Valentine, B. (2012). A critical examination of popular assumptions about the benefits and outcomes of monogamous relationships. *Personality and Social Psychology Review, 17,* 124–141.

Conlon, J. (1995). Why lovers can't be friends. In R. M. Stewart (Ed.), *Philosophical perspectives on sex and love* (pp. 295–300). New York: Oxford University Press.

Cook, M., and McHenry, R. (1978). *Sexual attraction.* Oxford: Permagon Press.

Crouse, B. B., and Mehrabian, A. (1977). Affiliation of opposite-sexed strangers. *Journal of Research in Personality, 11*, 38–47.

Darwin, C. (1871). *The descent of man, and selection in relation to sex* (Vol. 2). London: John Murray.

Demir, M., and Doğan, A. (2013). Same-sex friendship, cross-sex friendship, personality and happiness: A cross-cultural comparison. In F. Sarracino (Ed.), *The happiness compass: Theories, actions and perspectives for well-being. Psychology of emotions, motivations and actions* (pp. 67–90). Hauppauge, NY: Nova Science.

Dixon, D. (1983). Erotic attraction to amputees. *Sexuality and Disability, 6*, 3–19.

Dixson, B. J., Dixson, A. F., Bishop. P. J., and Parish, A. (2010). Human physique and sexual attractiveness in men and women: A New Zealand–U.S. comparative study. *Archives of Sexual Behavior, 39*, 798–806.

Dixson, B. J., Dixson, A. F., Li, B., and Anderson, M. J. (2007). Studies of human physique and sexual attractiveness: Sexual preferences of men and women in China. *American Journal of Human Biology, 19*, 88–95.

Domhoff, G. W. (2003). *The scientific study of dreams: Neural networks, cognitive development and content analysis*. Washington, DC: American Psychological Association.

Doskoch, P. (1995). The safest sex. *Psychology Today, 28*, 46–49.

Ebbeson, E. B., Kjos, G. L., and Konečni, V. J. (1976). Spatial ecology: Its effects on the choice of friends and enemies. *Journal of Experimental Social Psychology, 12*, 505–518.

Erlandsson, K., Nordvall, C. J., Öhman, A., and Häggström-Nordin, E. (2012). Qualitative interviews with adolescents about "friends-with-benefits" relationships. *Public Health Nursing, 30*, 47–57.

Feinberg, D. R., Jones, B. C., Little, A. C., Burt, D. M., and Perrett, D. I. (2005). Manipulations of fundamental and formant frequencies influence the attractiveness of human male voices. *Animal Behaviour, 69*, 561–568.

Feingold, A. (1991). Sex differences in the effects of similarity and physical attractiveness on opposite-sex attraction. *Basic and Applied Social Psychology, 12*, 357–367.

Feinman, S., and Gill, G. W. (1978). Sex differences in physical attractiveness preferences. *Journal of Social Psychology, 105*, 43–52.

Festinger, L., Schachter, S., and Back, K. (1950). *Social pressures in informal groups: A study of human factors in housing*. Stanford, CA: Stanford University Press.

Flora, C. (2010, November 1). The puzzle of pretty boys. *Psychology Today*. Retrieved September 20, 2013, from http://www.psychologytoday.com/articles/201012/the-puzzle-pretty-boys

Fouts, H. N., Hallam, R. A., and Purandare, S. (2013). Gender segregation in early-childhood social play among the Bofi foragers and Bofi farmers in Central Africa. *American Journal of Play, 5*, 333–356.

Freese, J., and Meland, S. (2002). Seven tenths incorrect: Heterogeneity and change in the waist-to-hip ratios of Playboy centerfold models and Miss America Pageant winners. *Journal of Sex Research, 39*, 133–138.

Freud, S. (1900). The interpretation of dreams (first part). In J. Strachey (Ed.), *The standard edition of the complete psychological works of Sigmund Freud* (Vol. 4, pp. 1–338). London: Hogarth Press and the Institute of Psycho-analysis (1986).

Freud, S. (1905a). Three essays on the theory of sexuality (6th ed.). In J. Strachey (Ed.), *The standard edition of the complete psychological works of Sigmund Freud* (Vol. 7, pp. 125–243). London: Hogarth Press and the Institute of Psycho-analysis (1986).

Freud, S. (1905b). Fragment of analysis of a case of hysteria. In J. Strachey (Ed.), *The standard edition of the complete psychological works of Sigmund Freud* (Vol. 7, pp. 7–122). London: Hogarth Press and the Institute of Psycho-analysis (1986).

Geher, G. (2012). Perceived and actual characteristics of parents and partners: A test of a Freudian model of mate selection. *Current Psychology, 19*, 194–214.

Giles, J. (2004). *The nature of sexual desire.* Westport, CT: Praeger.

Giles, J. (2010). Naked love: The evolution of human hairlessness, *Biological Theory*, *5*, 1–11.

Gilligan, C. (1982). *In a different voice: Psychological theory and women's development*. Cambridge, MA: Harvard University Press.

Glassenberg, A. N., Feinberg, D. F., Jones, B. C., Little, A. C., and DeBruine, L. M. (2010). Sex-dimorphic face shape preference in heterosexual and homosexual men and women. *Archives of Sexual Behavior, 39*, 1289–1296.

Goffman, E. (1959). *The presentation of self in everyday life.* New York: Anchor.

Halatsis, P., and Christakis, N. (2009). The challenge of sexual attraction within heterosexuals' cross-sex friendship. *Journal of Social and Personal Relationships, 26*, 919–937.

Hall, C. S. (1951). What people dream about. *Scientific American, 184*, 5, 60–63.

Hall, C. S. (1963). Strangers in dreams: An empirical confirmation of the Oedipus complex. *Journal of Personality, 31*, 336–345.

Hall, C. S., and Van de Castle, R. L. (1966). *The content analysis of dreams*. New York: Appleton-Century-Crofts.

Hansen, C., Rasmussen, C. C., Kløvedal, S. F. H., and Hendrich, S. (2014). *Utraditionelle kærlighedsforholder i et monogamtpræget samfund* (*Untraditional love relationships in a monogamous society*), Master's project, Roskilde University, Roskilde, Denmark.

Harvey, V. (2004). Constructing myths to manage romantic challenge in cross-sex friendships. In P. M. Backlund and M. R. Williams (Eds.), *Readings in gender communication*. Belmont, CA: Wadsworth/Thomas Learning.

Hatfield, E., and Berscheid, E. (1974). A little bit about love: A minor essay on a major topic. In T. Huston (Ed.), *Foundations of interpersonal attraction* (pp. 355–381). New York: Academic Press.

Hatfield, E., and Sprecher, S. (1986). *Mirror, mirror: The importance of looks in everyday life*. Albany: SUNY.

Hatfield, E., and Walster, G. W. (1981). *A new look at love*. Reading, MA: Addison-Wesley.

Hazan, C., and Diamond, L. M. (2000). The place of attachment in human mating. *Review of General Psychology, 4*, 186–204.

Hensley, W. E. (1994). Height as a basis for interpersonal attraction. *Adolescence, 29*, 469–474.

Hess, E. H. (1965). Attitude and pupil size. *Scientific American, 212*, 46–54.

Hicks, T. V., and Leitenberg, H. (2001). Sexual fantasies about one's partner versus someone else: Gender differences in incidence and frequency. *Journal of Sex Research, 38*, 43–50.

Hinz, V. B. (1989). Facial resemblance in engaged and married couples. *Journal of Social and Personal Relationships, 6*, 223–229.

Honneth, A. (2013). *Freedom's right: The social foundations of democratic life*. New York: Columbia University Press.

Hupka, R. (1981). Cultural determinants of jealousy. *Alternative Lifestyles, 4*, 310–315.

Jacklin, C. N., and Maccoby, E. E. (1978). Social behavior at thirty-three months in same-sex and mixed-sex dyads. *Child Development, 49*, 557–569.

Kaggwa, A. (2013, June 13). When men, women want more than "just friends." *Observer* (Uganda). Retrieved August 3, 2014 from http://www.observer.ug/

Keiser, S. (1953). A manifest Oedipus complex in an adolescent girl. *Psychoanalytic Study of the Child, 8*, 99–107.

Keller, K. (2007). *Cultures of infancy*. New York: Psychology Press.

Kenrick, D. T., Groth, G. E., Trost, M. R., and Sadalla, E. K. (1993). Integrating evolutionary and social exchange perspectives on relationship: Effects of gender, self-appraisal, and involvement level on mate selection criteria. *Journal of Personality and Social Psychology, 64*, 951–969.

Kinsey, A. C., Pomeroy, W. B., and Martin, C. E. (1948). *Sexual behavior in the human male*. Philadelphia: W. B. Saunders.

Kinsey, A. C., Pomeroy, W. B., Martin, C. E., and Gebhard, H. (1953). *Sexual behavior in the human female*. Philadelphia: W. B. Saunders.

Knapp, M. L., Hall, J. A., and Horgan, T. G. (2013). *Non-verbal communication in human interaction* (8th ed.). New York: Cengage Learning.

Krafft-Ebing, R. von. (1997). *Psychopathia sexualis* (D. Falls, Trans.). London: Velvet (Original work published 1886).

Kuhl, P. K. (1991). Human adults and human infants show a "perceptual magnet effect" for the prototypes of speech categories, monkeys do not. *Perception & Psychophysics, 50*, 93–107.

Langlois, J. H., Kalakanis, L., Rubenstein, A. J., Larson, A., Hallam, M., and Smooth, M. (2000). Maxims or myths of beauty? A meta-analytic and theoretical review. *Psychological Bulletin, 196*, 390–423.

Langlois, J. H., Roggman, L. A., Casey, R. J., Ritter, J. M., Reiser-Danner, L. A., and Jenkins, V. Y. (1987). Infant preferences for attractive faces: Rudiments of a stereotype? *Developmental Psychology, 23*, 363–369.

Lazarsfeld, P., and Merton, R. K. (1954). Friendship as a social process: A substantive and methodological analysis. In M. Berger, T. Abel, and C. H. Page (Eds.), *Freedom and control in modern society* (pp. 18–66). New York: Van Nostrand.

Levine, T. R., and Mongeau, P. A. (2010). Friends with benefits: A precarious negotiation. In M. Bruce and R. M. Stewart (Eds.), *College sex—Philosophy for everyone: Philosophers with benefits* (pp. 91–102). Oxford: Wiley-Blackwell.

Lisk, R. D., and Baron, G. (1982). Female regulation of mating location and acceptance of new mating partners following mating to sexual satiety: The Coolidge effect demonstrated in the female golden hamster. *Behavioral and Neural Biology, 36*, 416–421.

Little, A. C., DeBruine, L. M., and Jones, B. C. (2014). Sex differences in attraction to familiar and unfamiliar opposite-sex faces: Men prefer novelty and women prefer familiarity. *Archives of Sexual Behavior, 43*, 973–981.

Little, A. C., Jones, B. C., and DeBruine, L. M. (2011). Facial attractiveness: Evolutionary based research. *Philosophical Transactions of the Royal Society B, 366*, 1638–1659.

Little, A. C., Penton-Voak, I. S., Burt, D. M., and Perrett, D. I. (2003). Investigating an imprinting-like phenomenon in humans: Partners and opposite-sex parents have similar hair and eye colour. *Evolution and Human Behavior, 24*, 43–51.

Lortie-Lussier, M., Cote, L., and Vachon, J. (2000). The consistency and continuity hypothesis revisited through the dreams of women at two periods of their lives. *Dreaming, 10*, 67–76.

Lu, X. (2010). Rethinking Confucian friendship. *Asian Philosophy, 20*, 225–245.

Maccoby, E. E. (1990). Gender and relationships: A developmental account. *American Psychologist, 45*, 513–520.

Madrigal, L., and Kelly, W. (2007). Human skin-color sexual dimorphism: A test of the sexual selection hypothesis. *American Journal of Physical Anthropology, 132*, 470–482.

Maltz, W., and Boss, S. (1997). *In the garden of desire: The intimate world of women's sexual fantasies*. New York: Broadway Books.

Maner, J. K., Kenrick, D. T., Becker, D. V., Delton, A. W., Hofer, B., Wilbur, C. J., and Neuberg S. L. (2003). Sexually selective cognition: Beauty captures the mind of the beholder. *Journal of Personality and Social Psychology, 6*, 1107–1120.

Marrow, J. (1997). *Changing positions: Women speak out on sex and desire*. Holbrook, MA: Adams Meida.

McGee, L. (2011). Benefits for divorcing women. Reader comment on A. Ben-Zeév (2011), In the name of love: Friends with benefits, *Psychology Today*. Retrieved October 13, 2014, from http://www.psychologytoday.com/blog/in-the-name-love/201109/friends-benefits/comments

Miller, A. (1969). Analysis of the Oedipal complex. *Psychological Reports, 24*, 781–782.

Miller, M. J., Denes, A., and Ranjit, Y. (2014). Touch attitudes in cross-sex friendships: We're just friends. *Personal Relationships, 21*, 309–323.

Millet, C. (2003). *The sexual life of Catherine M.* (A. Hunter, Trans.). London: Corgi.

Mongeau, P. A., Knight, K., Williams, J., Eden, J., and Shaw, C. (2013). Identifying and explicating variation among friends with benefits relationships. *Journal of Sex Research, 50*, 37–47.

Monsour, M. (1992). Meanings of intimacy in cross- and same-sex friendships. *Journal of Social and Personal Relationships, 9*, 277–295.

Monsour, M. (2002). *Women and men as friends: Relationships across the life span in the 21st century*. Mahwah, NJ: Lawrence Erlbaum Associates.

Montoya, R. M., and Horton, R. S. (2013). A meta-analytic investigation of the processes underlying the similarity-attraction effect. *Journal of Social and Personal Relationships, 30*, 64–94.

Montoya, R. M., Horton, R. S., and Kirchner, J. (2008). Is actual similarity necessary for attraction? A meta-analysis of actual and perceived similarity. *Journal of Social and Personal Relationships, 25*, 889–922.

Morris, P., White, J., Morrison, E., and Fisher, K. (2013). High heels as supernormal stimuli: How wearing high heels affects judgments of female attractiveness. *Evolution & Human Behavior, 34,* 176–181.

Morry, M. M. (2005). Relationship satisfaction as a predictor of similarity ratings: A test of attraction-similarity hypothesis. *Journal of Social and Personal Relationships, 22*, 561–584.

Morry, M. M. (2007). Relationship satisfaction as a predictor of perceived similarity among cross-sex friends: A test of the attraction-similarity model. *Journal of Social and Personal Relationships, 24*, 117–138.

Muirstein, B. I. (1972). Physical attractiveness and marital choice. *Journal of Personality and Social Psychology, 22*, 8–12.

Munroe, R. L., and Romney, A. K. (2006). Gender and age differences in same-sex aggregation and social behavior: A four-culture study. *Journal of Cross-Cultural Psychology, 37*, 3–19.

Myers, J. E., Madathil, J., and Tingle, L. R. (2005). Marriage satisfaction and wellness in India and the United States: A preliminary comparison of arranged marriages and marriages of choice. *Journal of Counseling and Development, 83*, 183–190.

Nettle, D. (2002). Women's height, reproductive success and the evolution of sexual dimorphism in modern humans. *Proceedings of the Royal Society London, B, 269*, 1919–1923.

New York Times Magazine (2000, May 7). The way we live poll. *New York Times Magazine*, 76, 20–132.

Nietzsche, F. (2007). Nachgelassene fragmente 1876 gruppe 23. *Digitale Kritische Gesamtausgabe Werke und Briefe* [Posthumous fragments 1876 group 23. *Digital critical edition of the complete works and letters*]. Retrieved October 12, 2014, from http://www.nietzschesource.org/#eKGWB/NF-1876,23[72]

Nikolajeva, N. (2014, February 21). Er der dig? Amalie faldt for fyr i toget [Is it you? Amalie fell for a fellow on the train]. *Metroxpress*, 2.

Nisbett, R. E., and Wilson, T. D. (1977). The halo effect: Evidence for unconscious alteration of judgment. *Journal of Personality and Social Psychology, 35*, 250–256.

O'Meara, J. (1989). Cross-sex friendship: Four basic challenges of an ignored relationship. *Sex Roles, 21*, 525–543.

Owen, J., Fincham, F. D., and Manthos, M. (2013). Friendship after a friends with benefits relationship: Deception, psychological functioning, and social connectedness. *Archives of Sexual Behavior, 42*, 1443–1449.

Paine, R. (1969). In search of friendship: An exploratory analysis in "middle-class" culture. *Man, 4*, 505–524.

Parten, M. (1932). Social participation among preschool children. *Journal of Abnormal and Social Psychology, 28*, 136–147.

Paul, E. L., McManus, B., and Hayes, A. (2000). "Hookups": Characteristics and correlates of college students' spontaneous and anonymous sexual experiences. *Journal of Sex Research, 37*, 76–88.

Pelham, B. W., Carvallo, M., and Jones, J. T. (2005). Implicit egotism. *Current Directions in Psychological Science, 14*, 106–110.

Penton-Voak, I. S., and Perrett, D. I. (2000). Female preference for male faces changes cyclically: Further evidence. *Evolution and Human Behavior, 21*, 39–48.

Perrett, D. I., Lee, K. J., Penton-Voak, I., Rowland, D., Yoshikawa, S., Burt, D. M., . . . Akamatsu, S. (1998, August 27). Effects of sexual dimorphism on facial attractiveness. *Nature, 394*, 884–887.

Pollick, F. E., Kay, J. W., and Heim, K. (2005). Gender recognition from point-light walkers. *Journal of Experimental Psychology, 31*, 1247–1265.

Poulsen, F. O., Holman, T. B., Busby, D. M., and Carroll, J. S. (2012). Physical attraction, attachment styles, and dating development. *Journal of Social and Personal Relationships, 30*, 301–319.

Rawlins, W. K. (1982). Cross-sex friendship and the communicative management of sex-role expectations. *Communication Quarterly, 30*, 343–352.

Reddy, V. (2010). Engaging minds in the first year: The developing awareness of attention and intention. In J. G. Bremner and T. D. Wachs (Eds.), *The Wiley-Blackwell handbook of infant development* (2nd ed.) (Vol. 1, pp. 365–393). Oxford: Wiley-Blackwell.

Reeder, H. M. (2000). "I like you . . . as a friend": The role of attraction in cross-sex friendships. *Journal of Social and Personal Relationships, 17*, 329–348.

Rose, S. (1985). Same- and cross-sex friendships and the psychology of homosociality. *Sex Roles, 12*, 63–74.

Rose, A., and Rudolph, K. D. (2006). A review of sex differences in peer relationship processes: Potential trade-offs for the emotional and behavioral development of girls and boys. *Psychological Bulletin, 132*, 98–131.

Rubenstein, A. J., Kalakanis, L., and Langlois, J. H. (1999). Infant preferences for attractive faces: A cognitive explanation. *Developmental Psychology, 35*, 848–855.

Rubin, K. H., Bulkowski, W. M., and Parker, J. G. (2006). Peer interactions, relationships, and groups. In W. Damon, R. M. Lerner, and N. Eisenberg (Eds.), *Handbook of child psychology: Vol.3. Social, emotional, and personality development* (6th ed., pp. 571–645). New York: Wiley.

Rubin, L. B. (1985). *Just friends: The role of friendship in our lives*. New York: Harper and Row.

Rubin, Z. (1980). *Children's friendships*. Cambridge, MA: Harvard University Press.

Sartre, J.-P. (1956). *Being and nothingness: An essay on phenomenological ontology* (H. E. Barnes, Trans.). New York: Philosophical Library (Original work published 1943).

Schneider, A., and Domhoff, G. W. (2014). DreamBank. Retrieved June 12, 2014, from http://www.dreambank.net/

Schredl, M. (2012). Continuity in studying the continuity hypothesis of dreaming is needed. *International Journal of Dream Research, 6*, 114–124.

Schredl, M., Desch, S., Röming, F., and Spachmann, A. (2009). Erotic dreams and their relationship to waking-life sexuality. *Sexologies, 18*, 38–43.

Seiden, A. M., and Bart, P. B. (1975). Woman to woman: Is sisterhood possible? In N. Glazer-Malbin (Ed.), *Old family/new family: Interpersonal relationships* (pp. 122–151). New York: Van Nostrand.

Shakespeare, W. (2003). *Romeo and Juliet*. Retrieved November 5, 2014, from http://pages.towson.edu/quick/romeoandjuliet/rnjtext.htm#Act 2

Singh, D. (2006). Universal allure of the hourglass figure: An evolutionary theory of female physical attractiveness. *Clinics in Plastic Surgery, 33*, 359–370.

Slater, A., Von der Schulenburg, C., and Badenoch, M. (1998). Newborn infants prefer attractive faces. *Infant Behavior and Development, 21*, 345–354.

Spock, B. (1967). *Baby and child care*. New York: Pocket Books.

Stass, J., and Willis, F. (1967). Eye contact, pupil dilation, and personal preference. *Psychonomic Science, 7*, 375–376.

Stephens, W. O. (2010). What's love got to do with it? Epicureanism and friends with benefits. In M. Bruce and R. M. Stewart (Eds.), *College sex: Philosophy for everyone: Philosophers with benefits* (pp. 77–90). Oxford: Wiley-Blackwell.

Symons, D. (1979). *The evolution of human sexuality*. New York: Oxford University Press.

Tlachi-Lópeza, J. L., Eguibar, J. R., Fernández-Guasti, A., and Lucio, R. A. (2012). Copulation and ejaculation in male rats under sexual satiety and the Coolidge effect. *Physiology & Behavior, 106*, 626–630.

Tomlinson, N., Hicks, R., and Pellegrini, R. (1978). Attributions of female college students to variations in pupil size. *Bulletin of the Psychonomic Society, 12*, 477–478.

Tucker, J. (2008, October 18). The friends who become lovers. *Telegraph*. Retrieved May 10, 2014, from http://www.telegraph.co.uk/education/3357237/The-friends-who-become-lovers.html

Underwood, M. K. (2003). *Social aggression among girls*. New York: Guilford Press.

VanderDrift, L. E., Lehmiller, J. J., and Kelly, J. R. (2010). Commitment in friends with benefits relationships: Implications for relationship and safe-sex outcomes. *Personal Relationships, 19*, 1–13.

Vātsyāyana. (1994). *The complete Kāma Sūtra* (A. Danielou, Trans.). Rochester, VT: Park Street Press.

Vigil, J. M. (2007). Asymmetries in the friendship preferences and social styles of men and women. *Human Nature, 18*, 143–161.

Walster, E., Aronson, V., Abrahams, D., and Rottmann, L. (1966). Importance of physical attractiveness in dating behavior. *Journal of Personality and Social Psychology, 4*, 508–516.

Weaver, A., MacKeigan, K. L., and MacDonald, H. A. (2011). Experiences and perceptions of young adults in friends with benefits relationships: A qualitative study. *Canadian Journal of Human Sexuality, 20*, 41–51.

Weinberg, M. S., Williams, C. J., and Pryor, D. W. (1995). *Dual attraction: Understanding bisexuality* (Reprint edition). Oxford: Oxford University Press.

Werking, K. (1997). *We're just good friends: Women and men in nonromantic relationships*. New York: Guilford Press.

White, G. L. (1980). Physical attractiveness and courtship progress. *Journal of Personality and Social Psychology, 39*, 660–668.

Whiting, B. B., and Edwards, C. P. (1988). *Children of different worlds: The formation of social behavior*. Cambridge, MA: Harvard University Press.

Wiggins, J. S., Wiggins, N., and Conger, J. C. (1968). Correlates of heterosexual somatic preference, *Journal of Personality and Social Psychology, 10*, 82–90.

Williams, O. (1944). The leg in the subway. In C. Aiken (Ed.), *A comprehensive anthology of American poetry* (pp. 456–457). New York: Modern Library.

Willis, J. T. (2014). Partner preferences across sexual orientation and biological sex. *Personal Relationships, 21*, 150–167.

Wilson, J. R., Kuehn, R. E., and Beach, F. A. (1963). Modification in the sexual behavior of male rats produced by changing the stimulus female. *Journal of Comparative and Physiological Psychology, 56*, 636–644.

Wiszewska, A., Pawlowskia, B., and Boothroyd, L. G. (2007). Father-daughter relationship as moderator of sexual imprinting: A facialmetric study. *Evolution and Human Behaviour, 28*, 248–252.

Xiaohe, X., and Whyte, M. K. (1990). Love matches and arranged marriages: A Chinese replication. *Journal of Marriage and the Family, 52*, 709–722.

Zilbergeld, B. (1999). *The new male sexuality* (Rev. ed.). New York: Bantam.

Index

acceptance, 88, 115
accessories, 8
acquaintanceship, 83–84. *See also* stranger/strangers: change into acquaintance
admiration, 4, 26
adoptive relations. *See* kinship
aesthetically pleasing, 3, 24, 32
affiliation, 2, 3, 4, 19, 21–22, 203. *See also* affiliative attraction
affiliative attraction, 22
Alice's Adventures in Wonderland, 178
Allure, 27
allure, 25–33; meaning of, 32; near magnetic quality, 28; origin, 33–43; representations of oneself, 30; three interrelated features, 28. *See also* baring and caressing: goal of allure; being drawn; cross-sex friend/cross-sex friendship: allure; helplessness; intimately joined/intimate joining: feature of fantasy of allure; physical appearance: allured by; physical attraction: component of forms of interpersonal attraction; physical attraction: no allure; romantic partner/partners: allure; sexual friend/sexual friendship: allure; sexual interaction: awareness taken up in allure; sexual partner/sexual partners: allure; sexual partner/sexual partners: romantic allure; stranger/strangers: allure; stranger/strangers: alluring person
America, 130
American Beauty, 26–27
anal intercourse, 20
anallingus, 21
anus, inserting fingers into, 147
anxiety, 42, 112
Aristotle, 21, 86–87, 88, 168
assumption of similarity, 5
athletic ability, 3
autochthonic. *See* sexual fantasy/fantasies: autochthonic

back arching, 7, 8
ballet, 8
baring. *See* baring and caressing
baring and caressing, 4–5, 9, 180, 190, 191; conjoining of bodies, 170; exchange of, 192; goal of allure, 154, 156; heterosexual same-sex friends lack desires, 85, 93; infant-parent, 93; physical expression of vulnerability and care, 145; romantically attracted to, 171;

baring and caressing (*cont.*)
sexual attraction, 172. *See also* sexual desire: baring and caressing core components; sexual partner/sexual partners: baring body to
Barker, Meg, 149
bathing, 30
Beatles, 2
Beijing, 185
being drawn, 28–29, 33, 54, 56, 160, 201; attraction of friendship, 159, 162; contacted stranger, 60–63; cross-sex friends, 120–122, 125; fantasy, 32; romantic attraction, 194–196, 198; sense of helplessness, 31; sexual experience, 142; sexual friends, 155–156, 158; unnoticing stranger, 55, 60. *See also* allure
belly, 18, 36
belly dancing, 8
Beske-Rechek, April, 109
Biellmann spin. *See* ladies' figure skating
bisexual/bisexuals, 46, 149–150, 180–181, 182; attraction, 46
body in motion, 6
bonding, 92
Boys and Girls, 86
breast-feeding, 93
breasts, 8, 36, 64, 79, 134, 142, 150, 161; fondling and sucking, 20, 21; male preference, 36–37; sucking, 147. *See also* breast-feeding; Venus or Woman of Willendorf
Buddha, Gautama, 42
buttock/buttocks, 5, 6, 7, 8, 24, 59; male preference, 36–37. *See also* caress/caressing: buttocks; Venus or Woman of Willendorf

car, 10, 13
cardinal principle of dating, 18
caress/caressing, 5, 9, 30, 145, 153; automated quality, 142; buttocks, 134; cared for by, 152, 170; degrees of, 135; intimate, 45, 84; meanings, 197; melt under, 161; mutual, 199; naked skin, 20, 21, 134; of the penis, 145; through clothing, 135; of the vagina, 145; while having sex, 142. *See also* baring and caressing
cartoon, 12
catwalk, 8
celebrities, 2
charm, 26
Christakis, Nicolas, 117–118
classmates, 1, 201
close relationships, 84, 97
clothes/clothing, 8, 9, 27; designer, 9. *See also* fetishism; figure: women's clothing emphasizes; sexual fantasy/fantasies: clothing
companionate love. *See* love: companionate
companionship. *See* friendship: companionship
Confucius, 88
Conlon, James, 178–179
constancy, 88, 115, 180
Coolidge effect. *See* sexual interaction: Coolidge effect
couples, 85
courting, 166
cross-sex friend/cross-sex friendship, 106; allure, 118–125; ambivalence, 121; American and Turkish, 88; attraction of friendship, 121; becomes sexual friendship, 135–136; "Can men and women be just friends?," 111, 113, 116; China, 85–86; deny sexual attraction, 102–104; different from homosexual friendships, 100; does not involve a sexual relationship, 99; emotional support for males, 101; fall in love, 184–189; female experience, 105–106; gender differences, 108–111; Greece, 85; guilt or anxiety, 112; intentions, 112; jealous partner, 104; little scholarly attention, 99; male motives, 100–101; men glimpse world through female eyes, 101; not allowed in oppressive and religious regimes, 85; open and honest, 116; in popular films, 86; public relations challenge, 102; romantic partner, 197; safety, 123;

seen as preliminary to a romantic or sexual relationship, 86; sex gets in the way, 113; sexual arousal, 107, 108; sexual attraction, 101–104; sexual attraction a burden, 104, 111, 121, 204; sexual attraction as motivational/foundational element, 116–118, 141; situation dramatically changed, 85; touching, 107–108; Ugandan view, 106; United States, 85; warm and protective environment, 120; women criticized for, 102; women validate self-image, 106. *See also* helplessness: cross-sex friend; romantic partner/partners: apprehensive about cross-sex friend; sexual intercourse: with cross-sex friend; sexual relationship/relationships: cross-sex friendships not involving; sexual relationship/relationships: cross-sex friendships preliminary to; stranger/strangers: difference from cross-sex friend
cunnilingus, 20

da Vinci, Leonardo, 119
daydreaming, 48
Derailed, 56
descriptions: dreams, 78; experience of sexual attraction, 31
disliking, 2, 87, 183–184
Domhoff, G. William, 75
Doskoch, Peter, 31
dreams, 71–81; characters in, 94; images, 94. *See also* father/fathers: alluring dream stranger for female; father/fathers: in dreams; Freud, Sigmund: latent dream thoughts; Freud, Sigmund: manifest dream content; Freud, Sigmund: theory of dream interpretation; mother/mothers: alluring females in men's dreams; mother/mothers: in dreams
Dual attraction: Understanding bisexuality, 149

ear. *See* tongue: pressing into ear
Egypt, 58
ejaculation, 65, 157, 194. *See also* sperm
embarrassment/embarrassed, 143, 144, 204
embrace/embracing, 28, 69, 124, 136, 142, 150, 173, 191, 193; arousing, 161; intimate, 173; naked, 125, 150, 155, 193; naked and passionate, 134; sensual, 20, 21
emotional closeness, 152
encouraging, 12
enticement, 26
eye contact, 47–52, 58–64, 69; infant, 80
eye lids, 58
eye liner, 58
eye makeup, 58
eyes, 4, 13, 17, 48–49, 51, 58–60, 155; basic feature of sexual attraction, 58; color of ocean, 75; glistening, 58; inviting, 63; joy in her, 76; photographs motionless, 67; sparkle with liking of friendship, 197; women's eyes larger than men's, 58. *See also* eye contact; eye lids; eye liner; eye makeup; eye shadow; irises; mascara; pupils; whites of eyes
eye shadow, 58

Facebook, 132
face/faces, 24; averageness, 42; father's, 35; infant's preference for attractive, 41–42; opposite-sex, 28; shape, 5; women's, 42
familial relations. *See* kinship
"familiarity breeds contempt," 183
family, 3, 35, 71, 80, 92, 101; Western nuclear, 80. *See also* kinship
family friends, 1
father/fathers, 37–38, 71; adoptive, 34; alluring dream stranger for female, 74, 75–76; boy attempts to affiliate to and learn from, 80; in dreams, 71, 73–76, 77–79; early father–daughter relationship, 93; females more ambivalent relationship with, 73; little girl's feelings transferred to, 34; male authority figure, 73–74; male plays father-like role for girl, 80; takes on a sexual attractiveness for girl, 74;

father/fathers (*cont.*)
threatens to take the mother away, 73; women attracted to faces similar to, 35; women's image of their father's body, 35. *See also* stranger/strangers: father as an intruding; stranger/strangers: father symbolized as aggressive
fear of rejection, 16, 17
fellatio, 5, 20. *See also* touching: in fellatio
fetishism, 24; clothing, shoes, or handbags, 24
figure: curvaceous, 36; hourglass, 27, 35, 36, 59; ideal female, 35; male preference varies, 36; pear-shaped, 36; women's clothing emphasizes, 8
financial resources, 3
fingers, 9, 32, 148, 149, 161. *See also* anus: inserting fingers into; vagina: inserting fingers into
"flovers," 128
foot/feet, 8, 28, 56
fore-pleasure, 157, 194
Franklin, Benjamin, 184
free association, 73, 79
freedom, 61; to choose friends, 85; in fantasies, 31; sexual attraction's, 21
free will, 29, 201–203. *See also* freedom
Freud, Sigmund, 34, 38, 72, 157; latent dream thoughts, 72; manifest dream content, 72; theory of dream interpretation, 72
friendship, 2, 3–4, 83–99, 86–99; adolescence, 91; adulthood, 92; children's, 91; Chinese ideas, 88; companionship, 87–88, 105, 115, 119, 120, 132, 174–178, 197; enjoyment of company, 87–88, 90, 96, 115, 119; factor of gender, 91–92; formation, 25; question of erotic component, 84; reciprocity, 87, 88, 115; same-sex, 84–88, 91–93, 99–101, 117, 129, 151–152, 169; Scottish moral philosophers, 87; well-wishing and well-doing, 86–88, 115, 119–120, 146, 155, 159, 196. *See also* acceptance; acquaintanceship; Aristotle; constancy; cross-sex friend/cross-sex friendship; homosexual/homosexuals: same-sex friendships; honesty; loyalty; openness; sexual friend/sexual friendship; trust; understanding
Friends with Benefits, 129
friends with benefits, 128, 131, 132. See also *Friends with Benefits*; sexual friend/sexual friendship
FWB, 132, 140. *See also* friends with benefits
FWB relationship. *See* sexual friend/sexual friendship

gait, 7, 8
gaze, 6, 25, 29, 48, 49, 61; helpless before, 158; mutual, 47, 48; sexual attraction, 61
geishas, 8
gender/genders: appropriate, 41, 45, 49; basis of bisexual attraction, 149–150; completed by something it lacks, 149; desired, 23; in friendship, 91; friendship not dependent on, 169; in homosexual interaction, 149; merging with, 148, 150; in romantic attraction, 181; transgender and intersex, 174. *See also* cross-sex friend/cross-sex friendship: gender differences; friendship: factor of gender; gender isolation; romantic partner/partners: sex (gender) important; sexual fantasy/fantasies: gender differences; sexual friend/sexual friendship: gender imbalance in expectations; touch: gender differences
gender isolation, 183; breaking out of, 147–148; leads to sexual attraction, 185; loss of, 149; overcoming, 149, 180; ultimate pull of romantic attraction, 185
genitals, 21; changes in, 25; rubbing together, 20
Gilligan, Carol, 101
Goffman, Erving, 52

"Gold digger prank!," 10
gold diggers, 11
golden hamster, 66
good-looking, 78, 79
good smelling, 7, 18
guilt/guilty, 22, 38, 74, 112, 113, 143, 144, 204

hair, 5, 6, 9, 18, 32, 37, 64, 67, 155, 161; body, 60; red, 6; scent of, 123. *See also* hairstyles
hairstyles, 27
Halatsis, Panayotis, 117–118
Hall, Calvin, 73, 74, 79
hand/hands, 6, 17, 18, 181, 190; hand-holding, 9, 32, 192, 195, 197; holding breast, 161; holding vulva, 161; intervene in sex with, 158; on legs, 77, 78; shaking, 134; touches, 122, 188, 190–192; under clothing, 145
Hatfield, Elaine, 177
heart rate, 25
height, 18–19, 39
helplessness, 28, 29, 31, 32, 54, 201; challenges sense of free will, 201–205; cross-sex friend, 120–123, 125; eye contact, 60, 61; after having sex, 143; romantic allure, 194–196; seen-before stranger, 65; sexual friends, 156–160, 162; unnoticing stranger, 55. *See also* allure; gaze: helpless before; sexual relationship/relationships: helplessness in
Hendrix, Jimi, 167
heterosexual attraction, 205. *See also* sexual attraction
heterosexual friendships. *See* cross-sex friend/cross-sex friendship; friendship: same-sex; intimacy: women's same-sex friendships; sexual desire: in same-sex heterosexual friendships; sexual friend/sexual friendship
high heels, 7–8
high-status others, 2
hip/hips, 6, 7, 9, 36, 155; shaking, 8
homosexual attraction, 27, 150, 205
homosexual/homosexuals, 23–24, 39, 46, 85, 105, 147; same-sex friendships, 100, 152. *See also* homosexual attraction; homosexual interaction; homosexuality; lesbian/lesbians
homosexual interaction, 147, 149
homosexuality, 27, 84, 182–183
honesty, 88, 115
Honneth, Axel, 87
hookup/hookups. *See* sexual friend/sexual friendship: not serial hookup; sexual intercourse: hookups; stranger/strangers: hooking up
hourglass figure. *See* figure: hourglass
hug/hugging, 93, 104, 123, 124, 135, 142, 162

implicit egoism, 39
impression formation, 5
inbreeding, 38
infant, lack of communication skills, 34. *See also* baring and caressing: infant-parent; eye contact: infant; face/faces: infant's preference for attractive; infantile fantasies; mother/mothers: alluring for female infant; mother/mothers: infant's awareness of; mother/mothers: relation to female infant; romantic love: beginnings in mother-infant relationship; sexual desire: beginnings in the mother-infant relationship; sexual fantasy/fantasies: infantile fantasies
infantile fantasies, 137
intelligence, 3; no predictive value, 15
interpenetration, 150
interpersonal attraction, 1–43, 196, 203, 204; positive attitude toward another person, 2; two-dimensional model, 4
intersex. *See* gender/genders: transgender and intersex
intimacy, 45, 110, 123, 151, 178, 190; cross-sex friendship, 107–108; fantasies of, 203; fantasized sexual, 69; female emotional ties, 92; of friendship, 83, 84; physical, 33, 45–46, 53, 54, 63, 69, 118; psychological,

intimacy (*cont.*)
172–173, 180, 191, 195; in sex leads to friendship, 153; sexual friendships, 152; women's same-sex friendships, 151. *See also* intimately joined/intimate joining; romantic attraction: psychological intimacy and showing concern; sexual interaction: intensity and physical intimacy
intimately joined/intimate joining, 30–33, 63, 119, 156, 163, 173, 192; fantasized, 57; feature of fantasy of allure, 193; goal of allure, 189; image, 160
irises, 58–59

Japanese culture, 8, 166
jealous/jealousy, 102, 105, 114, 131, 139–140, 141, 151. *See also* cross-sex friend/cross-sex friendship: jealous partner; romantic partner/partners: jealous

Kāma Sūtra, 9, 16–17
kimono, 8
kin, 12
kindness, 12
kinship, 2, 3; adoptive relations, 3; familial relations, 3
kissing: erotic, 20, 30; passionate, 20; vulva, 193. *See also* leg/legs: kisses; romantic attraction, embracing, kissing, or being physically intimate; tongue: deep kissing

ladies' figure skating, 8; Biellmann spin, 8; layback, 8
layback. *See* ladies' figure skating
"Leg in the Subway," 56
leg/legs, 36, 52, 56–57, 78; caressed, 77; crosses in an alluring way, 119; inadvertently pressing, 64; kisses, 78; licking, 56–57; nylon-encased, 56; quicken steps, 155; rest head on, 103, 104; wrapping around, 150, 155. *See also* thighs
lesbian/lesbians, 24, 105
level of aspiration, 16, 17
lifelong partners, 1, 205
light-point displays, 8
liking, 2, 13, 86, 87; acquaintances, 83–84; attraction of, 121; different from romantic attraction, 169–170; of friendship, 172, 196, 197, 198; friendship includes, 3; glistening eyes signal, 58; increased, 70; seek out company, 197, 203; spending time together encourages, 183–184; touching expresses, 122. *See also* mutual liking
lips, 9, 32, 78, 142, 148, 161, 192
long-term partner, 14–15
long-term relationship/relationships, 16, 17, 60; women socialized to consider, 68
love, 2, 3; between friends, 133; brother and sister, 133; companionate, 177; mother and child, 133. *See also* romantic love
love at first sight, 19, 21, 168, 181, 190, 191
love at many sights, 19
loyalty, 88, 115, 116, 159, 180

maikos, 8
makeup, 27. *See also* eye liner; eye makeup; eye shadow; mascara
making love/make love, 63, 69, 128
manipulation, 16
marital status, 30
marriage/marriages, 97–99, 130, 177, 189; arranged, 98; blind, 98; distinct from friendship, 98–99, 177; free-choice, 98; friendships are more important, 98; importance of friendship, 177; loveless, 190; Nietzsche on, 177; proper place for having sex, 130; unhappy marriages, 177. *See also* marital status
mascara, 58
masturbated by one's partner, 20
masturbating one's partner, 20
matching hypothesis, 16–17, 34, 40, 167

metaphysical isolation, 95; attempt to overcome, 138, 147, 155; child's idea of, 96–97; different from romantic attraction, 180, 185; friendship lessens sense of, 101; fundamental motive for friendship, 96, 118, 155; sexual friendship, 162. *See also* mutual liking: overcoming metaphysical isolation
metaphysics, 95
midriff. *See* Venus or Woman of Willendorf
Millet, Catherine, 148
Miss America pageant winners, 36
Mona Lisa, 119–120
money, 10, 11, 13
Mongeau, Paul, 132
mother/mothers, 36–38; adoptive, 40; alluring females in men's dreams, 74, 76–78, 79; alluring female strangers a copy of, 79; alluring for female infant, 80; alluring stranger, 79; children strongly attracted and attached, 73; in dreams, 71, 74, 76–78, 79; fantasized biological, 41; first stranger, 79; infant's awareness of, 79–80; men choose women who resemble, 35; primary care giver, 34, 93; relation to female infant, 80–81; wanting to be, 166; warmth of skin, softness of breasts, succulence of smell, 79–80. *See also* love: mother and child; romantic love: beginnings in mother-infant relationship; sexual desire: beginnings in the mother-infant relationship; stranger/strangers: mother prototypical
mouth, 6, 148, 149, 150, 155
musical abilities, 21
mutual liking, 3, 90, 96, 101, 120; with acquaintance, 83; between a man and a woman, 99–100; close to another awareness, 180; companionship, 174, 197; compliments alluring sense of being drawn, 121; of friendship, 198; friendship based on, 86; hallmark of friends, 176; intimate warmth, 106; natural connection to sexual relationship, 100; overcoming metaphysical isolation, 184; of sexual friendship, 154; without unpleasantness of rivalries, 105
mutual vulnerability and care, 172, 175, 176, 197. *See also* baring and caressing: physical expression of vulnerability and care; romantic love: mutual vulnerability and care; unpleasantness: vulnerability and care
My Best Friend's Wedding, 86

naked fondling, 30. *See also* breasts: fondling and sucking
neck, 6, 9, 32, 161, 197
neonate, 79
Nietzsche, Friedrich. *See* marriage/marriages: Nietzsche on
No Strings Attached, 129

Oedipal complex, 34, 73, 74
O'Meara, J. Donald, 102
one-night stand, 130
openness, 88, 115, 176, 178
opposite-sex parent, 34, 35, 37–41, 73–74, 78–81, 93, 108, 202
optimal breeding, 38
oral-anal interaction, 20. *See also* anallingus
oral-oral interaction, 20. *See also* kissing
orgasm/orgasms, 30; multiple, 157
overall size of the figure, 36
overweight, 22

partners in friendship love, 128
pear-shaped figure, 36
penis, 20, 148–149, 150, 158, 181. *See also* sexual intercourse: caresses of the penis; sexual intercourse: vagina takes in an envelops penis
peripheral-vision contact, 47, 49, 50
personality/personality traits, 4, 17–23, 52–53, 59, 171–172; attributing, 5; clothes imply, 8; correlated with sexual preferences, 37; no predictive value, 15; sexual attraction not directed to,

personality/personality traits (*cont.*) 12–13; unknown, 6. *See also* romantic partner/partners: personality/personality traits; sexual partner/sexual partners: personality traits; similarity: personality
perspiration, 25
phatic communication, 69
physical appearance, 6–25, 26–27, 33–34, 36, 39, 42–43, 58, 67; allured by, 119, 155, 191; change perception of, 70; touching as observation of, 122
physical attraction: component of forms of interpersonal attraction, 3–4; formation of friendships, 25; no allure, 26, 28, 33; nonsexual, 24; not the same as sexual attraction, 23, 32, 33; origin, 41–43; tied to human appearance, 24
physical unattractiveness/physically unattractive, 12, 24, 22; lack of youth, lack of health, oncoming death, 42; origin of idea of, 42; sexually attractive, 24
Playboy centerfold, 36
pleasure, 21; erotic, 157; fore-pleasure, 157, 194; friendship, 88; peak, 157, 194; of release, 157; sexual, 30
polyamory/polyamorous relationships, 139, 179
Polynesian culture, 140
possessions, 9, 10, 11, 13, 168
pretending to be ill, 17
problem of other minds, 96
proximity, 4, 25, 52, 68, 91, 97, 184
psychoanalytic investigations, 35
pupils, 47, 48, 58, 59–60

reciprocity, 52; inherent in romantic love, 171, 177. *See also* friendship: reciprocity
renaissance masters. *See* Rubens, Peter Paul; Titian
romantic attraction, 20; allure, 189–199; apparently romantic relationships, 167–168; being attracted to one's real or potential love, 168; cannot be defined in terms of enjoyment, 175; companionship, 175; continuous fantasizing, 169; dependent on gender, 169; difference from sexual attraction, 168; driven by sexual attraction, 173; embracing, kissing, or being physically intimate, 173–174, 178, 191–192, 195; not an intense liking, 169; not part of sexual attraction, 168; psychological counterpart to sexual attraction, 171; psychological intimacy and showing concern, 172; relationship with friendship, 180, 184–189; in *Romeo and Juliet*, 175–177; sexual attraction integral part of, 20–21; stranger, 21; varying degrees, 171; volatility and swiftness of onset and decline, 169; vulnerability and care, 171–172. *See also* being drawn: romantic attraction; gender/genders: in romantic attraction; gender isolation: ultimate pull of romantic attraction; liking: different from romantic attraction; metaphysical isolation: different from romantic attraction; romantic love: difference from romantic attraction; romantic love: fundamentally connected to romantic attraction
romantic love, 2, 19, 97–98, 128, 133, 170, 178, 179, 181; beginnings in mother-infant relationship, 93; close ties to sexual attraction, 165; commitments not always part of, 134; complaints raised in, 141; difference from romantic attraction, 165–166; fundamentally connected to romantic attraction, 166; mutual vulnerability and care, 176, 177; not distinct from sexual relationship, 108; not experienced in an emotional way, 188; not part of sexual desire, 138; not part of sexual interaction, 138; periods where unclear, 172; in *Romeo and Juliet*, 175–177, 178, 181, 190, 191–192, 195; sense of merging, 138; sexual attraction part of, 20; swift in its onset, 172. *See also* companionate love; reciprocity: inherent in romantic

love; sexual desire: intimate part of romantic love; sexual relationship/relationships: romantic love not distinct from
romantic partner/partners, 9, 29, 54, 103, 201; actual or potential sexual partner, 174; allure, 189–199; also friends, 172, 178; apprehensive about cross-sex friend, 109–110; brought closer by having sex, 153; choosing, 188; in dreams, 71; fears loss of the other, 175; friends become, 127; intimate exchanges, 170; jealous, 192, 114; need not be friends, 174; one's friend, 97; open psychologically and emotionally, 170; ostensible, 166–167; personality/personality traits, 168–169, 171–172; possible/potential, 166, 168, 181, 186; role of sexual attractiveness, 108; sex (gender) important, 174; sharing personal feelings, 170; show desired care, 171; spend time together, 183–184; supportive, 102; usual partners for sex, 130; vulnerable before, 171. *See also* sexual attraction; trust: romantic partners
romantic relationship, 22
Romeo and Juliet. *See* romantic love: in *Romeo and Juliet*
Rubens, Peter Paul, 36
Rubin, Lillian, B., 89, 93, 136–137

safety, 88, 115, 116. *See also* cross-sex friend/cross-sex friendship: safety
saliva, 56, 57, 147
Sartre, Jean-Paul, 61
Schneider, Adam, 75
Scottish moral philosophers. *See* friendship: Scottish moral philosophers
self-confidence, lack, 22
self-deception, 10, 11, 143
self-disclosure, 52, 91, 92, 176
self-esteem, 21
self-loathing, 38
sense of familiarity, 51, 68, 198–199
sense of humor, 12, 21
sex organs, 148, 158. *See also* penis; vagina; hand/hands: holding vulva; kissing: vulva
sexual activity/activities, 138, 169, 182; attraction leads to, 115; fantasies, 30, 196; renewal, 65; resume, 66. *See also* sexual interaction
sexual attraction, 1–43; major role in people's lives, 1; social, behavioral, biological, and experiential components, 25–26. *See also* baring and caressing: sexual attraction; cross-sex friend/cross-sex friendship: sexual attraction; cross-sex friend/cross-sex friendship: sexual attraction a burden; cross-sex friend/cross-sex friendship: sexual attraction as motivational/foundational element; descriptions: experience of sexual attraction; freedom: sexual attraction's; gaze: sexual attraction; gender/genders: basis of bisexual attraction; gender isolation: leads to sexual attraction; heterosexual attraction; homosexual attraction; personality/personality traits: sexual attraction not directed to; physical attraction: not the same as sexual attraction; romantic attraction: difference from sexual attraction; romantic attraction: driven by sexual attraction; romantic attraction: not part of sexual attraction; romantic attraction: psychological counterpart to sexual attraction; romantic attraction: sexual attraction integral part of; romantic love: close ties to sexual attraction; romantic love: sexual attraction part of; sexual desire: distinct from sexual attraction; sexual interaction: basis in sexual attraction
sexual desire, 113, 122, 143, 152, 190; baring and caressing core components, 93; beginnings in the mother-infant relationship, 93; distinct from friendship, 93; distinct from sexual attraction, 27–28; intimate part of

sexual desire (*cont.*)
romantic love, 138; in same-sex heterosexual friendships, 84

sexual fantasy/fantasies, 29–31, 55, 149, 173, 194; autochthonic, 31, 201; brief and fleeting, 31; clothing, 145; concrete images, 46; contacted stranger, 55, 57–58, 62; faceless persons, 30; feature of allure, 28, 31–33, 54, 63, 195, 201, 203; friendship, 119–120, 123–125, 142–143; gender differences, 31; infantile fantasies, 137; masturbation, 190; romantic allure, 198; romantic partner/partners, 169, 173–174, 189–191, 193, 195–196; sexual friends, 160–162; stranger, 124, 191; unnoticing, 55–57. *See also* allure; being drawn: fantasy; freedom: in fantasies; infantile fantasies; intimacy: fantasies of; intimacy: fantasized sexual; intimately joined/intimate joining: fantasized; romantic attraction: continuous fantasizing; sexual activity/activities: fantasies; sexual intercourse: fantasy/fantasize; sexual intercourse: most usual fantasy; sexual partner/sexual partners: fantasize; sexual partner/sexual partners: sexual fantasies; touching: fantasizes

sexual friend/sexual friendship, 9, 107, 125, 128, 129; allure, 153–163; Canadian university students, 131; contentious, 136; crossed over into a romantic relationship, 169; cultural norms, 131, 139, 179; divorced persons, 131–132; films, 129; gender imbalance in expectations, 141; negative aspects, 140–141; negative views of, 136–140; not in China, 130; not serial hookup, 146; positive aspects, 140, 141; quality, 136; romantic expectations, 152; romantic relationships, 141; sex enriched friendship, 144; similar problems to romantic relationships, 141; similar to romantic partners, 153; students in Australia, 131; students in Denmark, 131; students in United Kingdom, 131; Swedish adolescents, 131; two paths to mutual closeness, 150–151; what counts as sexual friendship, 132–136

sexual images, 31

sexual immaturity, 7

sexual interaction, 20, 21, 30, 31, 45, 124, 134–138, 145–163; awareness taken up in allure, 193–194; basis in sexual attraction, 107; Coolidge effect, 66–67; in *The Crying Game*, 182; early physical interactions, 34; end of, 143–144; façades difficult to maintain, 144; fantasy of, 196; fundamental reason for, 93, 177; homosexual, 149; imagined, 69, 125; intensity and physical intimacy, 53; men and women friends without, 112, 115; romantic attraction, 195; romantic relationship, 189. *See also* anal intercourse; anus: inserting fingers into; breasts: fondling and sucking; caress/caressing: buttocks; cunnilingus; embrace/embracing; fellatio; gender isolation: breaking out of; gender isolation: loss of; gender isolation: overcoming; genitals: rubbing together; hug/hugging; masturbated by one's partner; masturbating one's partner; naked fondling; oral-anal interaction; oral-oral interaction; sexual intercourse; tongue: deep kissing; tongue: licking leg; tongue: pressing into ear; touching: extensive mutual; touching: sexual; vagina: inserting fingers into

sexual intercourse, 5, 20, 26, 30, 134, 147, 190; allure after, 109; caresses of the penis, 145; caresses of the vagina, 145; with cross-sex friend, 107; exchange male and female essences, 149; fantasy/fantasize, 55, 57, 124, 125; "having sex," 134; hookups, 132; most usual fantasy, 29; with several men, 80; sex organs helpless before

each other, 158; sex organs merging, 148; sexual friends, 155; vagina takes in an envelops penis, 150
sexual partner/sexual partners, 66, 108, 115, 116, 124; allure, 109, 189; baring body to, 170–171; cannot be friends, 129; childhood impulses, 35; choice, 18, 35, 37; drawn toward, 160; fantasize, 30, 124, 162; friend, 155; larger or taller, 7; loss of interest, 143; personality traits, 14, 190; returning to, 163; romantic allure, 195; romantic partner, 107, 174, 186; sex important, 174; sexual fantasies, 160; similar appearance to self, 37, 39; similarity of appearance, 39; vulnerable to, 170
sexual relationship/relationships, 112–113, 117; helplessness in, 194; preclude best part of friendship, 137, 140; problems, 151–152; romantic love not distinct from, 108; stigma for women, 109; touching in, 107; unwanted, 204; with "true friends," 133, 147. *See also* close relationships; cross-sex friend/cross-sex friendship: does not involve a sexual relationship; cross-sex friend/cross-sex friendship: seen as a preliminary to a romantic or sexual relationship; long-term relationship/relationships; mutual liking: natural connection to sexual relationship; romantic love; romantic partner/partners; sexual friend/sexual friendship; sexual interaction; sexual partner/sexual partners
Shakespeare, William, 175, 184
shame/ashamed, 38, 74, 131, 143
shared activity/activities, 88, 90, 91, 92, 97, 151, 176, 178, 180, 115, 197
shoes, 8, 24, 56. *See also* fetishism: clothing, shoes, or handbags; high heels
short-term partner, 15
siblings, 3
similarity: affect interpersonal attraction, 3; personality, 14, 17
Sinatra, Frank, 62
skin, 5; color, 19; darker-pigmented, 19; fairer, 19; "good enough to eat," 9; natural object of the caress, 135; smooth, 143; soft and smooth, 122; texture, 123. *See also* caress/caressing: naked skin; mother/mothers: warmth of skin
smell, 6–7, 18, 79, 142, 184. *See also* hair: scent of
smile/smiling, 6–7, 9, 63, 67, 76, 169; *Mona Lisa*, 119; ritualistic acknowledgement, 84; sign of friendship, 155; support sexual intent of eye contact, 62
social media, 132
solipsism, 95
spending time together, 84, 138, 183–185. *See also* liking: spending time together encourages
sperm, 65, 147, 148, 149
Spock, Benjamin, 79
status, 9, 10, 14; social, 10; social or economic, 9. *See also* high-status others
stereotyping, 5
stomach: butterflies in, 171; fire in, 186, 188, 189, 198, 199; flat, 8
"Strangers in the Night," 62
stranger/strangers, 5, 6, 14, 21, 22, 43; allure, 53–71; alluring person, 81; change into acquaintance, 71; contacted, 47, 49–50, 51; difference from acquaintance, 83–84; difference from cross-sex friend, 106–107, 121; in dreams, 71–81; father as an intruding, 73; father symbolized as aggressive, 74; hooking up, 132; interacted-with, 51–52, 84; mother prototypical, 79; no such thing as seen-before, interacted-with, 52, 53; partner for sex, 130; romantically attractive, 191–192; seen-before, 50, 138; seen-before contacted, 51, 64; seen-before unnoticing, 51, 64–65; unknownness, 45, 46, 54, 62, 123; unnoticing, 46–47, 48, 49, 50, 51, 190. *See also* being drawn: contacted

stranger/strangers (*cont.*)
stranger; being drawn: unnoticing stranger; father/fathers: alluring dream stranger for female; helplessness: seen-before stranger; helplessness: unnoticing stranger; mother/mothers: alluring female strangers a copy of; mother/mothers: alluring stranger; romantic attraction: stranger; sexual fantasy/fantasies: stranger; sexual fantasy/fantasies: unnoticing
subculture, 8
support, 88, 115, 116, 176, 180; emotional, 92, 100–101, 105, 146, 152, 185, 188
supportive, 12, 102, 122, 156, 171, 196; emotionally, 185
"swept off one's feet," 28

"tall, dark, and handsome," 18, 19
Taoist philosophy, 149
taste, 6, 45, 142, 149
teeth, 9, 45
The Crying Game, 181. *See also* sexual interaction: in *The Crying Game*
"The Myth of Love at First Sight," 20
The Nature of Sexual Desire, 145
The Odyssey, 179
theory of mind, 96
thighs, 6, 9, 32, 64, 104; male preference, 36–37
Titian, 36
Todas of India, 140
tongue, 148, 149, 150; deep kissing, 147; licking leg, 56–57; pressing into ear, 147
touch, 6, 50, 107, 162, 175, 192; friendly, 122; frequently, 124; gender differences, 107–108; helpless, 158; sexual, 122; sexual attraction through, 64. *See also* touching
touching, 25, 34, 52, 69, 107, 122, 127, 142; clothed, 162; extensive mutual, 159; fantasizes, 191, 195; in fellatio, 149; flirtatious, 107, 124, 127, 135; friendly, 122; hands, 181; sexual, 107, 122, 124, 127, 135, 162. *See also* physical appearance: allured by; physical appearance: touching as observation of; sexual relationship/relationships: touching in
train, 6
transgender. *See* gender/genders: transgender and intersex
trust, 75, 76, 88, 115, 137, 140, 159; romantic partners, 170

unconscious: consideration, 111; desire, 72; impulse or idea, 38; intensions, 113; level of awareness, 38, 95
understanding, 88, 115, 180
undressing, 30
unkind, 12
unknownness. *See* stranger/strangers: unknownness
unpleasantness: feelings, 112; not inherent in sexual attraction, 204; rivalries, 105; vulnerability and care, 175
Up in the Air, 129
upper-body side-sway, 7

vagina, 20, 147–149, 158, 182; inserting fingers into, 147. *See also* sexual intercourse: caresses of the vagina; sexual intercourse: vagina takes in and envelops penis
vaginal secretions, 147, 149
Vātsyāyana, 17, 157, 163
Venus, Cupid, Bacchus, and Ceres, 36
Venus or Woman of Willendorf, 35–36
voice/voices, 7, 68; higher-pitched female, 7; lower-pitched male, 7
vulva, 161. *See also* hand/hands: holding vulva; kissing: vulva

waist. *See* waist-to-hip ratio
waist-to-hip ratio, 36
"Waiting for Mr. Right," 188
walking, 5–6; stylized, 50; way of, 5, 7
Walster, G. William, 177
warmth, 34, 56; of friendship, 83, 84, 96, 106, 120–121, 123, 125, 132
way of dressing, 6

wealth, 9, 11, 168
wedding, 98, 175, 186, 187, 188, 189. See also *My Best Friend's Wedding*
well-being, 205
well-wishing and well-doing. *See* friendship: well-wishing and well-doing
Werking, Kathy, 139
Western culture, 7, 80, 85, 86, 98, 104, 110. *See also* family: Western nuclear; sexual friend/sexual friendship: cultural norms
When Harry Met Sally, 86, 113, 116
whites of eyes, 58, 59, 60
"Why lovers can't be friends," 178
Williams, Oscar, 56
women's facials, 9
work colleagues, 1, 185, 201

"You Really Got a Hold on Me," 2

About the Author

James Giles was born in Vancouver, Canada, and studied at the University of British Columbia and the University of Edinburgh, where he gained a PhD in philosophy. He is adjunct professor of psychology at Roskilde University, Denmark, and a lecturer at the University of Cambridge, Institute for Continuing Education. Dr. Giles has taught at universities in Europe, the UK, Hawaii, Guam, and Australia, and has traveled widely through Asia and the Pacific. Among his writings are *The Nature of Sexual Desire*, *No Self to Be Found: The Search for Personal Identity*, and *A Study in Phenomenalism.* For more information, visit www.james-giles.com.